Marijuana
Medical
Handbook

Marijuana Medical Handbook

A Guide to Therapeutic Use

Ed Rosenthal

Tod Mikuriya, M.D.

Dale Gieringer

QUICK AMERICAN ARCHIVES

Published by Quick American Archives
Oakland, California

Publisher's Cataloging in Publication
(Prepared by Quality Books Inc.)

Rosenthal, Ed.
    Marijuana medical handbook / Ed Rosenthal, Tod Mikuriya, Dale Gieringer.
      p.   cm.
    Includes bibliographical references and index

      1. Marijuana 2. Marijuana—Health aspects. I. Mikuriya, Tod H. II. Gieringer, Dale H. III. Title.
RM666.C266R68 1997   615'.323962
                                       QBI97-40161

Project Manager: Andrew McBeth
Cover and Photography Conversion: Larry Utley
Marijuana Leaf on Cover: André Grossman
Editing: Judith Abrahms, Liz McBeth
Layout: Nancy Koerner
Illustrations: Chris Peterson
Indexer: Trisha Lamb Feuerstein

Printed in the U.S.A. by Publisher's Express

Acknowledgments

All the patients and caregivers who shared their knowledge.

Lynne Barnes, R.N.

Valerie and Mike Corral

Everyone who worked and voted for Proposition 200
and Proposition 215.

Gordon Farrel-Ethridge

Tom Flowers

Jon Gettman

HEMP B.C.

John Morgan, M.D.

Dennis Peron

Debora Zippel

EYES OF THE WORLD

Wake up to find out that
you are the eyes of the world,
and the heart has its beaches
its homeland and
thoughts of its own;
wake now, discover that
you are the songs that
the morning brings,
but the heart has its seasons,
its evenings
and songs of its own.

Words by Robert Hunter of The Grateful Dead

Table of Contents

Appendices

Preface

Marijuana is one of the most benign and effective medicines used by humankind. The government has banned its use for various political and social reasons. In spite of this, millions in the U.S. seek relief through the use of this herb.

The *Marijuana Medical Handbook* is a "hands-on" guide to the use of marijuana medically. It is written for current users as well as for people who have never used before. The information in this book is unavailable from any other source.

About the Authors

Ed Rosenthal is the bestselling author of many books about marijuana, its use, and its cultivation. He has been writing the popular "Ask Ed" column in *High Times* magazine for many years. He is a member of the International Cannabis Research Society and an adviser to the San Francisco Cannabis Cultivator's Club, formerly the San Francisco Cannabis Buyer's Club.

Dale Gieringer, Ph.D., is the coordinator of California National Organization for the Reform of Marijuana Laws (NORML), where he has sponsored research and publications on the uses of marijuana, including *Marijuana, Driving and Accident Safety, Health Tips for Marijuana Smokers,* and a marijuana-smoking filtration device study.

"In my years with NORML, I have spoken with hundreds of patients who use marijuana as medicine," says Dr. Gieringer. "The multifarious experiences, diagnoses, and reactions they have reported provide an invaluable basis for this book."

Dr. Tod Mikuriya is a practicing psychiatrist with over 30 years of clinical experience in the medical use of cannabis. He is the author of *Marijuana: Medical Papers* and served as a director of marijuana research for the National Institute of Mental Health in 1967.

Introduction

This book was inspired by a visit to my mother at her retirement community in Florida. She was having a get-together for many of her friends. One fellow was undergoing radiation therapy for cancer. My mother's next-door neighbor was suffering from high intraocular pressure, which would eventually cause blindness from glaucoma. My mother suffered from arthritis and lack of appetite. One woman was telling her friend she suffered from insomnia. Two friends had spasms, one intestinal and the other in her limbs. All of them suffered from occasional or chronic depression.

I realized that every one of my mother's guests could benefit from marijuana. In traditional medicine, it would be the first drug prescribed for these ailments. The propaganda of the government had been so effective that no one there even suspected that they were being deprived of a very effective medicine that is also remarkably benign. Compared with the high-priced prescription drugs they were taking, with their notorious side effects, marijuana would be much safer.

However, in 1990 I was discouraged from even suggesting this medicine to these people who were suffering for the lack of it. The government had just shaken off the decades-old suit initiated by Robert Randall that had sought to have marijuana reclassified as an experimental drug.

President Clinton continued the vendetta. Operations against marijuana growers were stepped up. He initiated new criminal penalties; then his administration worked to suppress marijuana medical research.

In 1993, I learned of an organization in Baltimore, a buyers' club, that would supply marijuana to medical patients at reasonable prices. Soon Dennis Peron opened a buyers' club in San Francisco. Dennis's club was open until the State Attorney's Office raided it in July 1996. I went there one Tuesday and saw members receiving free small packages of marijuana. It was not of the best quality, but the packages contained usable amounts. I was impressed. Here was a person who ran a club that sold marijuana, giving it away to the needy. It was very moving. This man was showing more care and compassion than the entire medical establishment and the government combined.

I realized that outside of the few cities where buyers' clubs are functioning, there is no place for a person who needs marijuana to find it easily. Most people who need it for medical purposes do not know a dealer and have no access to one through their communities.

Usually, when a person needs medicine, s/he can obtain it. When a medicine is illegal, however, everything changes. The safety of the commercial marketplace disappears and is replaced by the corruption of the black market. Prices are high, quality and availability are variable, and there is no recourse for the patient who runs into a problem. The legal ramifications and threats to personal safety stemming from the purchase or even the simple possession of the herb can also be serious.

In 1994, about 2,000 people died from using aspirin. No deaths were reported from the use of marijuana. In fact, in the entire history of reporting on drug deaths in the U.S., not one fatality has ever been convincingly attributed to marijuana use. Ironically, then, the most harmful and dangerous aspect of marijuana use is government regulation.

The laws forbidding marijuana use for medical purposes constitute cruel and unusual punishment, inflicted on the victims of disease. Not only do they threaten people's safety and health; they limit marijuana's availability and keep its price high.

The best-quality marijuana sells for between $300 and $500 per ounce. If it were grown and sold in the same way as other herbs, an ounce would cost only a few dollars. At a time when health care costs are spiraling upwards, it is a shame that Americans do not have legal access to this remarkably economical medicine.

This book has been written and published to alleviate suffering. It describes the conditions for which marijuana has a beneficial effect, how marijuana can be obtained, how people can supply themselves reliably by growing a small garden, and how to use it medically.

— *Ed Rosenthal*

1

HOW SAFE IS MARIJUANA?

DOONESBURY
by Garry Trudeau

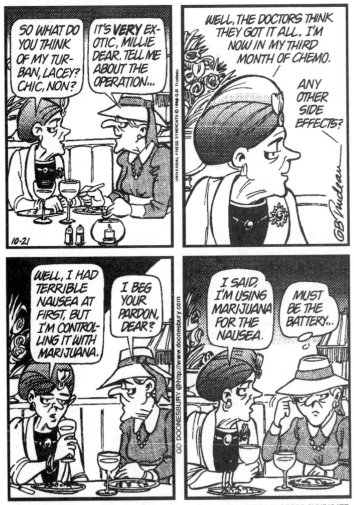

1

How Safe is Marijuana?

Marijuana is exceedingly safe. Drug Enforcement Agency (DEA) Administrative Judge Francis Young wrote, in his decision recommending legalization of medical marijuana, "Marijuana, in its natural form, is one of the safest therapeutically active substances known to mankind." Unlike other psychoactive drugs, including alcohol, aspirin, opiates, nicotine, and caffeine, it does not cause fatal overdoses. From animal experiments, it has been estimated that a lethal dose of cannabis would be 40,000 times a normal dose: approximately 40 pounds!

The government has never reported a death from cannabis use since it began keeping statistics. In 1993, the government's Drug Awareness Warning Network (DAWN) reported that a total of 29,200 people had reported using marijuana recently while appearing at an emergency clinic. This does not mean that the visit was caused by the use of marijuana. If there are 10 million users, who smoke every other day on the average, this comes to a scant .0016%-per-use chance that one of them will end up in an emergency room for any reason, even a bee sting or a toe infection.

What about people who drive and use marijuana? Aren't they at risk?

Here's what the U.S. National Highway Transportation Safety Administration (NHTSA) has to say in "Marijuana and Actual Driving Performance," a study conducted in the Netherlands, using various dosages of marijuana, on freeways and under urban driving conditions. Marijuana intoxication in drivers is "in no way unusual compared to many medicinal drugs." (Hindrik W. J. Robbe and James O'Hanion, "Marijuana and actual driving performance," published as *Department of Transportation Report #DOT HS 808-078*, 1996.)

Marijuana does have some effect on driving ability, but is "not profoundly impairing." (Hindrik W. J. Robbe and James O'Hanion, "Marijuana and actual driving performance," published as *Department of Transportation Report #DOT HS 808-078*, 1996.)

Unlike alcohol, which encourages risky driving, marijuana appears to produce greater caution, apparently because its users are more aware of their state and better able to compensate for it. (Hindrik W.J. Robbe and James O'Hanion, "Marijuana and actual driving performance," published as *Department of Transportation Report #DOT HS 808-078*, 1996.)

This is not to say that marijuana cannot have adverse effects. Like all drugs, marijuana can cause harm if taken in excess or abused. In addition, certain people simply respond poorly to marijuana, finding it more unpleasant than beneficial. But what's important is that people have access to accurate information about marijuana. Without information, how will they know whether it will benefit them, what dose they should take, and how they can gain access to a regular supply?

Marijuana, botanically known as cannabis, has been around for thousands of years. Its use, both medical and recreational, has been recorded for centuries. Until 1937, it was legal and was commonly prescribed medicinally in the U.S. Despite its prohibition, marijuana continues to be one of the most widely used drugs in America.

Cannabis has been known as a medicinal plant since ancient times. In China, it appears in the ancient medical classic, *Pen Ts~ao*, by the legendary emperor Shen-Nung, as a remedy for "gout, rheumatism, malaria, beriberi, constipation, and

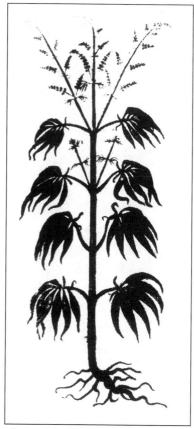

The first botanical illustration of Cannabis Sativa, dating from the first century A.D. From a manuscript of Dioscorides's Constantinopolitanus in the British Museum.

absent-mindedness." It was allegedly used by the famous surgeon Hua T'o to perform painless operations in the second century A.D. In the Roman world, cannabis was mentioned in the classic medical writings of Galen and Dioscorides, who imaginatively recommended the "juice of the seed" to prevent earaches and diminishing sexual desires, and flatulence. It was also regularly prescribed as a pain killer.*

The oldest archeological evidence of medical use of cannabis dates from the discovery, in 1994, in an Egyptian tomb of the third century A.D. In the tomb were the remains of a young girl who had died in childbirth, accompanied by traces of hashish, or concentrated cannabis resin, which had apparently been used to ease the difficulties of labor.

The medical properties of cannabis were brought to Europe in 1839 by an Irish physician, William B. O'Shaughnessy. He

* In fact, cannabis seeds have no medically active ingredients, though they have been used for human nutrition and animal feed since time immemorial. Hemp seed yields a nutritious edible oil that is high in linolenic acid and is also useful for cosmetic and industrial uses.

observed its use in India, then experimented with alcohol-based cannabis tinctures to treat rheumatism, rabies, cholera, tetanus, and convulsions. He described it as an analgesic and an "anti-convulsive remedy of the greatest value." In Victorian times, cannabis came to be popular in the treatment of painful menstruation and childbirth, asthma, migraines, neuralgia, and senile insomnia. By the late nineteenth century, however, its use began to wane as stronger and more conventional medicines became available.

Marijuana's use as a legal medicine was ended by a political misfortune. In 1937, the Marijuana Tax Act, a bill to ban marijuana, was brought before Congress. The director of the Federal Bureau of Narcotics, Harry Anslinger [who was, by the way, a former Prohibition official], led the attack on marijuana with bogus charges of violence that focused on Hispanics, African Americans and other minority groups.

One of the most vocal groups to oppose the bill was the American Medical Association (AMA). Dr. William Woodward, a member of the AMA, argued that cannabis was not dangerous and that its medicinal use would be severely curtailed by the proposed measures. The Prohibitionists prevailed through the use of a well-organized campaign of misinformation, and marijuana has been illegal in the U.S. ever since.

The Marijuana Tax Act of 1937 essentially ended the medicinal use of cannabis. In 1941, it was withdrawn from the U.S. pharmaceutical market because of public misconceptions and because of the burdensome paperwork imposed on pharmacists by law.

The medicinal value of marijuana was rediscovered during the recreational marijuana boom of the Sixties. In the early 1970s, it was reported that some young cancer patients found that smoking a joint could relieve the gut-wrenching nausea that resulted from chemotherapy. Clinical studies at Harvard and elsewhere soon confirmed marijuana's anti-nauseant properties.

W.B.OSHAUGHNESSY M.D.
Professor of Chemistry and Natural Philosophy.
Medical College Calcutta

Meanwhile, other patients were discovering that marijuana could help relieve glaucoma, chronic pain and muscle spasticity from spinal injuries and multiple sclerosis, and other complaints. Interest in the medical benefits of marijuana peaked in the late 1970s, when over 35 states passed legislation to establish medical marijuana research programs. Each program was eventually smothered by federal drug regulations, which made it virtually impossible to conduct scientific marijuana research.

Under the terms of the 1970 Controlled Substances Act, marijuana is classified as a Schedule 1 controlled substance, meaning that it has high abuse potential and no recognized medical use. Schedule 1 drugs cannot be used without explicit permission from the DEA and the Food and Drug Administration (FDA), which involves exhaustive paperwork, long delays, and almost certain refusal.

In 1972, the National Organization for the Reform of Marijuana Laws (NORML) petitioned the government to make marijuana a Schedule 2 drug. This action developed into a lawsuit that dragged on for 20 years and ended in defeat for NORML. In the meantime, frustrated patients were forced to seek other legal remedies.

In 1976, Robert Randall, a glaucoma patient, succeeded in persuading the federal government to supply him with marijuana under a new FDA "Compassionate Use" protocol. With the support of his physician, Randall, arguing that marijuana was the only drug that would prevent him from going blind, won a lawsuit against the federal government. The government grudgingly agreed to supply Randall with free marijuana from its own research farm in Mississippi. In later years, a dozen more patients managed to enroll in the Compassionate Use program, which required elaborate, time-consuming paperwork from their physicians. Pressed by a flood of new applicants who had been struck by the AIDS virus, the government closed the program to new applicants in 1991. Today, just eight patients receive marijuana legally in the U.S., for conditions including glaucoma, multiple sclerosis, epilepsy, and rare bone diseases.

In 1988, following extensive testimony, DEA Administrative Judge Francis Young ruled that marijuana's medical benefits were "clear beyond question" and that it should be reclassified as a Schedule 2 drug. Judge Young's recommendation was promptly overruled by DEA chief John Lawn, who, despite the fact that morphine and cocaine had earned a Schedule 2 classification, expressed concern that it would send the "wrong message" about marijuana's supposed harmfulness. After further legal twists and turns, the DEA ban was upheld by a federal appeals court in 1993. Hence, marijuana remains a Schedule 1 drug to this day.

Still, medical marijuana has attracted growing interest from health professionals. Although the AMA switched its position on marijuana after 1937, as it becomes more beholden to corporate interests, its California branch, the CMA, has called for research to establish guidelines for prescription use of cannabis. Other organizations, including the American Public Health Association, the Federation of American Scientists, the California Nurses' Association, the AIDS Life Lobby, and the AIDS Project-L.A., have been bolder in demanding outright legalization of medical marijuana.

In 1996, California and Arizona voters passed two state initiatives that recognized the value of marijuana for the sick. Exempting patients from prosecution for possessing or cultivating marijuana for medical use if they had a physician's recommendation. Now that Californians and Arizonans have approved these initiatives many hope that it will only be a matter of time before federal law is reformed to restore the right of U.S. citizens to use medical marijuana.

2

WHAT
MARIJUANA DOES

DOONESBURY
by Garry Trudeau

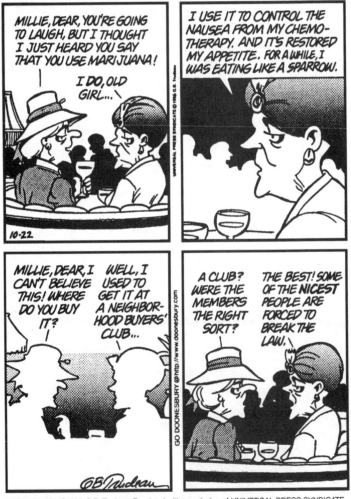

Panel 1: MILLIE, DEAR, YOU'RE GOING TO LAUGH, BUT I THOUGHT I JUST HEARD YOU SAY THAT YOU USE MARIJUANA!

I DO, OLD GIRL...

10-22

Panel 2: I USE IT TO CONTROL THE NAUSEA FROM MY CHEMO-THERAPY. AND IT'S RESTORED MY APPETITE. FOR A WHILE, I WAS EATING LIKE A SPARROW.

Panel 3: MILLIE, DEAR, I CAN'T BELIEVE THIS! WHERE DO YOU BUY IT?

WELL, I USED TO GET IT AT A NEIGHBORHOOD BUYERS' CLUB...

Panel 4: A CLUB? WERE THE MEMBERS THE RIGHT SORT?

THE BEST! SOME OF THE NICEST PEOPLE ARE FORCED TO BREAK THE LAW.

2

WHAT MARIJUANA DOES

Marijuana is primarily a psychoactive, or consciousness-altering, drug. Physically, its effects are modest and largely negligible. Marijuana's primary site of action is the brain, particularly the higher brain centers that affect consciousness. Receptors for marijuana are concentrated especially in the hippocampus, which affects the higher functions of feelings, memory, and action. By acting on these higher brain systems, marijuana produces some of its most striking medicinal benefits, affecting perception of pain, mood, hunger, and muscle control. Marijuana may also produce more subtle medical effects through direct action on bodily tissues, such as receptors in the immune system cells.

Marijuana users commonly report pleasurable sensations; after all, that's why people use it recreationally. There are also people who find it makes them uncomfortable. In practice, its effects on different people and in different circumstances vary, depending on individual temperament, physiology, mood, and the famous "set and setting" defined by Dr. Timothy Leary: the initial mindset of the user and the surroundings in which the user gets high.

Here are some of the more commonly reported impressions of "being high" on cannabis:

- Heightened attentiveness to sensory stimuli, especially touch, taste, and sound; heightened interest in food and in music.
- Free flow of ideas in rapid, loose, dreamlike succession; mild hallucinations with a "double consciousness" that some resemblances or connections are perceived, not real.

- Disruption of concentration and short-term memory.
- A sense of floating, light-headedness, or dizziness, and/or a sense of heaviness in the trunk and limbs.
- Hyperactivity, restlessness, hilarity, and talkativeness for the first hour or two, followed by sleepiness and/or torpor after two to six hours.
- Subjective "time expansion," a tendency to overestimate the amount of time that has passed.
- Impaired judgment and coordination, especially when performing complex tasks; confusion; difficulty expressing thoughts in words; slurred speech.

First-Time Use

The first use of marijuana is a special occasion. For reasons that aren't well understood, many people don't feel anything the first time they smoke it. They respond only the second or third time, as if it were necessary somehow to "prime" yourself for the experience. Some new users may actually act "stoned," but not notice it. The first-time threshold can usually be overcome by simply raising the dose. However, this greatly raises the risk of an unpleasant reaction. First-time users should proceed cautiously; they should be prepared to be incapacitated for a couple of hours.

Tolerance

Heavy marijuana users tend to develop a tolerance, or decreased sensitivity, to the effects of tetrahydrocannabinol (THC), the active ingredient in marijuana. Pleasant sensations such as euphoria tend to fade with heavy, regular use. On the other hand, the same may be true of undesirable effects, such as a rise in the heart rate (tachycardia).

Less frequently, patients may develop a tolerance to the medical benefits of marijuana. Sometimes this problem can be remedied by switching to a different variety or dosage method for a while.

DRUG INTERACTIONS

Marijuana rarely increases the toxic effects of other medicines. In this respect, it differs even from such common drugs as alcohol, which is extremely dangerous in combination with depressants, or aspirin, which is dangerous in combination with blood-thinning drugs such as coumarin. This is yet one more instance of marijuana's remarkable safety.

Certain drugs may interact with marijuana to stimulate tachycardia, among them the antidepressant nortriptyline, and possibly the popular stimulant and antiasthmatic ephedrine (an ingredient in so-called "herbal ecstasy" preparations). On the other hand, THC-induced tachycardia may be inhibited by beta blockers such as propranolol.

ADDICTIVENESS

Marijuana is not physically addictive. Smokers may use it many times daily for many years, then give it up with no difficulty. When a former user is asked how he or she quit, a typical reply is "I just didn't use it any more."

When experts compare marijuana with alcohol, nicotine, cocaine, opiates, caffeine, and other psychoactive drugs, they rank it at or near the bottom of the list in terms of dependence, reinforcement, and withdrawal potential. Still, like every human pleasure, the use of marijuana can be strongly habit-forming for a certain minority. About 10% of recreational users have trouble controlling their use. They are mostly troubled people who have difficulty with other drugs as well. A few drug treatment programs deal with marijuana abusers, but these make up a tiny proportion of the drug treatment clientele.

A minority of long-term, extremely heavy (several doses daily) recreational users experience subtle withdrawal symptoms when they give up marijuana. These include mild anxiety, depression, nightmares, difficulty sleeping, vivid dreams, irritability, tremors, perspiration, nausea, muscle convulsions, and restlessness. These symptoms, though mild, may persist for a few days, but are only noticeable in the heaviest abusers, and even then they present no real obstacle to anyone trying to quit.

PHYSICAL EFFECTS

Marijuana is exceedingly safe. This is not to say that marijuana cannot have adverse effects. Like all drugs, marijuana can be harmful if taken in excess or abused.

The effects of marijuana are experienced almost immediately after smoking. If it's taken orally, they're delayed an hour or more. When it is smoked, the effects are most pronounced for the first hour or two, declining gradually over the next three or four hours. They normally disappear after a good night's sleep. Unlike alcohol, opiates, cocaine, amphetamine, and many other drugs, pot doesn't produce unpleasant "hangover" or rebound effects—the high just fades away. A few supersensitive people may feel slightly sedated for a day or so after use.

Chronic users—those who smoke marijuana every day—may experience more prolonged, though low-level, effects, lasting days or even weeks after stopping. The reasons for this "cannabis haze" are uncertain.

One possible explanation is a buildup of residual cannabinoids in the system. THC is a highly fat-soluble drug that tends to be absorbed by fat tissues throughout the body. Most of the cannabinoids inhaled from a joint end up somewhere other than the brain. They are then slowly transferred back into the bloodstream over a period of many days. For occasional users, the blood concentration of residual THC is minuscule. However, chronic heavy use raises the level of residual THC to levels that can be detected for 48 hours or more.

THC has few noticeable physical effects on the body. The following symptoms are commonly reported:

- Dryness of the throat, resulting in thirst.
- Redness of the eyes' outer coating, or conjunctiva, due to dilation of the small blood vessels there.
- Speeding of the heartbeat, or tachycardia.
- Reduction of pressure inside the eye, a benefit for glaucoma patients.
- Dilation of the upper bronchial passages of the lungs.

In addition, marijuana smoke has irritating effects on the lungs, just like tobacco. These result not from cannabinoids, but from other, toxic byproducts of burning. Fortunately, they can be reduced by various smoke reduction methods, and completely eliminated by taking marijuana orally instead of smoking it.

CHEMICAL COMPOSITION OF MARIJUANA

The medicinal and psychoactive effects of marijuana are caused by a family of chemicals known as cannabinoids, which are present only in the marijuana plant. At least 61 cannabinoids have been identified in nature. Others have been chemically synthesized.

The main psychoactive ingredient in marijuana is delta-9-tetrahydrocannabinol, or THC [sometimes confusingly referred to as delta-1-THC under a different naming system]. However, other cannabinoids also have medicinal and/or psychoactive properties.

Cannabigerol (CBG), cannabichromene (CBC), cannabidiol (CBD), delta-8-THC, cannabicyclol (CBL), cannabinol (CBN), cannabitriol (CBT), cannabavarin (THCU), and other cannabinoids are among the various cannabinoids. All are known to have psychoactive or pharmacological effects. Because delta-9-THC is the major psychoactive ingredient in marijuana, it is regularly used to measure the herb's potency. Typical concentrations of THC are less than 0.5% for inactive hemp, 2% to 3% for marijuana leaf, and up to 4% to 8% for higher-grade seedless, or sinsemilla, bud. Higher concentrations can be found in extracts, tonics, and hashish (concentrated cannabis resin).

Therapeutic oral doses range from 2.5 to 20 milligrams of THC. A typical joint (1 gram of 2.5% leaf or 0.5 gram of 5% buds) contains 25 milligrams of THC. However, more than half this amount is normally lost in slipstream smoke, leaving the actual inhaled dose closer to 10 milligrams.

Experienced users have reported that different types of marijuana produce different highs and, medically, have different effects. Researchers theorize that the different proportions of cannabinoids in different varieties—or even different plant samples—create these varied effects.

MARIJUANA IN THE BODY

At the beginning of the 1990s, scientists learned that cannabinoids resemble a chemical that occurs naturally in the brain and that marijuana's effects are caused by biological mechanisms affected by this natural chemical.

The brain and nervous system contain many different systems of biological mechanisms, called receptor systems. Receptors are sites that react to specific chemicals and produce specific reac-

tions. The chemicals are called neurotransmitters, and the cas-
cade of chain reactions throughout the networks of these systems
is the process by which areas of the brain communicate with
each other; this is how the brain works. Most drugs produce their
effects by interfering with or activating the processes of specific
systems. Barbiturates, for example, have a nonspecific effect on
chloride ion channels; this increases the activity of a neurotransmitter called GABA; an increase in GABA activity has a sedative effect. Benzodiazepines, such as Valium®, have a specific
effect on receptor sites that increase GABA activity.

Before the discovery of a cannabinoid receptor system in the
early 1990s, some scientists speculated that marijuana produced its effects through nonspecific action, like barbiturates.
Nonspecific effects are generally broader and more dangerous
than the effects produced by receptor site activation.

In fact, marijuana's effects are produced by a cannabinoid
receptor system consisting of at least two cannabinoid receptor
types: CB1 and CB2, located in the brain and spleen, respec-
tively. The biological actions now associated with cannabinoid receptors include marijuana's effects as an analgesic, on
memory and cognition, on locomotor function, on endocrine
actions, and on other biological changes, including a decrease
in body temperature, changes in the heart rate, suppression of
nausea and vomiting, and decrease in intraocular pressure.
Scientists know to some degree how the CB1 receptors function, but have only a limited understanding of how canna-
binoceptive neurons interact with other neural systems. CB2
was discovered somewhat later than CB1, and knowledge of
CB2 is still slight.

Tolerance for marijuana develops from continued exposure
to large amounts of cannabinoids; in response, the brain
decreases the number of receptor sites available to bind

cannabinoids. When a heavy exposure ends, the receptor sites increase back to a natural level.

The naturally occurring neurotransmitter that the cannabinoid receptor system responds to is called anandamide (after the Sanskrit word for bliss). In its natural form, anandamide has a considerably lower potency than THC, the primary cannabinoid in marijuana. Yet anandamide does play an important role in the brain, and researchers at NIDA believe that they will be able to show that it helps the body cope with stress, pain, and nausea.

The locations of the cannabinoid receptors show continued promise for therapeutic research according to one prominent researcher at the National Institute of Mental Health (NIMH).

There are no reports of fatal cannabis overdose in humans. The safety reflects the paucity of receptors in medullary nuclei the part of the brain that controls respiratory and cardiovascular functions.

OVERDOSE AND TREATMENT

In a few cases, users may experience acute panic reactions, characterized by anxiety, paranoia, self-consciousness, loss of self-control, wild racing thoughts, and disorientation. Fortunately, such reactions are rare and usually subside within a couple of hours. No medical treatment is necessary. Sufferers should be reassured that their discomfort will be brief. Often, pleasant and unpleasant feelings occur in alternating waves, as thoughts ebb and flow.

Panic reactions are most likely to occur in novice users with excessive doses and in unpleasant surroundings. First-time users should take care to start with small amounts and to allow themselves ample comfort and time to experience the drug.

Occasionally, marijuana can produce unpleasant physical symptoms, including headaches, dizziness, nausea, and vomiting, which may be secondary to mental anxiety, and which are most common at heavy doses. A few individuals experience such symptoms regularly, like an allergic reaction. Most frequently, though, adverse physical reactions result from an overdose. Though never fatal, heavy overdoses are unpleasant and can be temporarily debilitating. Symptoms include anxiety, panic, excitement, hallucinations, and a racing heartbeat, proceeding to immobility, torpor, and unconsciousness. Fortunately, the effects are temporary and wear off after a few hours sleep. No antidote is needed.

Toxic overdoses occur less frequently with inhaled marijuana than with oral ingestion, because smokers can sense instantly when they have had enough or when the drug content is too high. At most, smokers may step "one toke over the line" before finding they are too high and stopping. Oral doses are much harder to gauge. It's easy to take a multiple dose of brownies and not know what's hit you until hours later.

Cannabis poisonings were more common around the turn of the century, when medicinal preparations were dispensed in potent tonics containing hundreds of doses per fluid ounce.

THE PARADOXICAL EFFECTS OF MARIJUANA

Marijuana has a "paradoxical" ability to produce precisely opposite reactions in different circumstances. Though it typically eases nausea, spasticity, pain, and insomnia, it can also aggravate them in exceptional situations or for exceptional subjects. Again, marijuana can cause euphoria, pleasure, or relaxation at one time and suffering, depression, or anxiety at another. The paradoxical nature of cannabis results from the fact that its effects are filtered through the highest centers of human consciousness. Thus the French poet Baudelaire called hashish "the mirror that magnifies," emphasizing the importance of personality as well as set and setting.

Marijuana appeals differently to different people. People who like it often use it to increase the intensity of their senses. They may smoke before eating, listening to music, watching plays or movies, or taking a walk or hike, or while spending time with others or just thinking. Many users report subjective feelings of creativity and inspiration, although these don't always stand up to later, sober analysis. Many devotees report feelings of euphoria, exhilaration, good will, empathy, and religious awe. They say marijuana helps them think about serious matters, to become introspective and spiritual, to get to the essence of things.

People who don't like marijuana complain of anxiety, self-consciousness, paranoia, social withdrawal, irritability, dysphoria, and loss of self-control. They may also find that it interferes with their ability to work, concentrate, and function.

SET AND SETTING

Marijuana's effects are especially responsive to variations in individual set and setting. Set is defined as what the user brings to the drug: his or her own medical situation, psychology, physiology, state of mind, and so on. Hence some patients are naturally more attuned to the therapeutic circumstances benefits of marijuana than others. Setting is the external situation in which the user takes the drug: the physical, sensory, and social environment. People who would normally find marijuana rewarding will often react unfavorably in the wrong circumstances, if they are pressed by obligations, discomfited by unpleasant company, or placed in disagreeable surroundings.

MARINOL®

One marijuana substitute is a synthetic drug, known as Marinol (whose generic name is dronabinol), which contains pure THC. Marinol was introduced to the market in 1986 as an antin-auseant for cancer chemotherapy. In 1993, it was also approved for nausea and appetite loss arising from AIDS wasting syn-drome. Both uses were approved by the FDA on the basis of controlled safety and efficacy studies.

At present, Marinol is marketed by the Unimed Corpor-ation. It is sold in the form of soft gel capsules containing syn-thetic THC dissolved in sesame oil, in doses of 2.5, 5, and 10 milligrams. Marinol is a Schedule 2 prescription drug (this is the most tightly controlled category).

The development of Marinol was promoted by federal offi-cials in the Reagan administration in the hope of stemming medicinal demand for crude cannabis. Its proponents argue that Marinol is preferable because it is a chemically pure pharmaceu-tical, produced in controlled doses, rather than a smoked herb, consisting of unknown quantities of different chemicals. In fact, Marinol has proven to be a poor and imperfect substitute for natural marijuana. Though some patients find it useful, many others report that it doesn't work as well as natural marijuana.

One possible limitation of Marinol is that it contains a sin-gle medically active cannabinoid, THC. It lacks other poten-tially active cannabinoids in natural marijuana, such as CBD. As we've seen, CBD may have unique medical benefits. As a result, pure THC may not be ideal for many patients.

Perhaps the greatest limitation of Marinol is that it comes only in oral doses. In contrast, natural marijuana can also be inhaled by smoking. Inhalation is preferable in many medical circumstances. In particular, chemotherapy patients are often so nauseated that they have trouble holding down any oral medication. The easiest way for such people to get marijuana into their systems is through inhalation.

Inhalation is also preferable when users need fast relief. Oral doses frequently take an hour or more to take effect, whereas inhaled marijuana takes effect almost at once. Patients can promptly treat a sudden attack of pain, or an oncoming seizure or muscle spasm, with smoked marijuana, but not with oral Marinol.

Another important advantage of inhalation is that it allows patients to regulate their dosage more accurately, through a process known as self-titration. Once you inhale marijuana, you can sense immediately whether it has had the effect you need. If not, you can just take another puff. With oral doses, however, you have to guess the proper amount beforehand, then wait an hour or so to see whether you were right. This makes it easy to overshoot or undershoot the mark.

All of this makes nonsense of claims by opponents of marijuana that only Marinol affords scientifically controlled, well prescribed dosages. For many purposes, such as relief of pain, discomfort, and nausea, patients are in a better position to adjust their own dose through self-titration than doctors who try to guess what oral dose is appropriate.

In fact, even though Marinol comes in well-defined doses, it may not be easy to predict how much of it will be absorbed into your system. This is because the bioavailability of oral THC varies greatly according to the state of your digestive system and other factors. The same oral dose may be insufficient on one occasion and overpowering on another. As a result, misdosage is a common problem with Marinol. In particular, patients appear to experience a high incidence of anxiety attacks due to overdose, a problem that may be aggravated by Marinol's lack of CBD.

Yet another major drawback of Marinol is its price, which is up to $300 per prescription. Patients can spend up to $4700 per month on Marinol. Unless you have good insurance, this is tough medicine. Marinol is so expensive because it's chemically synthesized. As we'll see, it's possible to produce high-potency extracts of THC much more cheaply from home-grown marijuana. When cannabis was still on the pharmaceutical market in the 1920s, a one-pint bottle containing 4700 doses could be bought for as little as $4, or one tenth of a cent per dose! In our own time, when the cost of health care is a major issue, it's ironic that our government has outlawed this uniquely affordable medication.

Marinol does have some advantages. It's medically pure, so there's no risk of contamination from bacteria, fungi, pesticides, or other contaminants that can creep into black-market marijuana.

In addition, Marinol doesn't involve the respiratory hazards of smoking. Of course, neither do oral preparations of natural cannabis. However, Marinol's consistency and purity have the advantage of predictability of strength when it is taken on a continuing basis. In contrast, homemade oral preparations often vary greatly in potency from batch to batch.

It's been suggested that pure THC should be better for smoking than natural marijuana because its vapors are free of the toxic pyrolytic compounds produced by burning leaf. It has been reported that some users open Marinol capsules and smoke the contents. Unfortunately, this practice can't be recommended, because Marinol is formulated with sesame oil, which produces a highly irritating smoke when burned.

The most important advantage of Marinol is its legality. Marinol can be prescribed by any physician who has a DEA license (most do). However, its use is tightly restricted by the fact that it's a Schedule 2 drug. Physicians frequently resist prescribing Marinol, especially when they must use triplicate prescription forms that can be monitored by the authorities. This can pose problems for patients who want it for conditions other than its FDA-labeled indications, namely cancer chemotherapy and AIDS.

In theory, any FDA-approved drug can be prescribed for any indication, whether it's mentioned on the label or not. However, the DEA has tried to subvert this principle in the case of Marinol. DEA regulations specifically warn that physicians who prescribe Marinol outside its approved uses of cancer chemotherapy and AIDS risk having their DEA licenses revoked and being criminally prosecuted (21 CFR Part 1308; *Federal Register* Vol. 51: 17477 (May 13, 1986)). Of the tens of thousands of prescription drugs approved by the FDA for sale in the U.S., Marinol is the only one to carry such a warning.

Fortunately, this regulation has not been enforced and there are serious questions as to its legality. In a 1992 letter to California NORML, Deputy Assistant Secretary of Health Dr. Jack Chow stated:

> "My staff has had several discussions with DEA on this issue . . . and we have been assured that as a matter of policy, DEA will not revoke a registration or take criminal action against a physician who prescribes Marinol for medical indications other than nausea associated with cancer chemotherapy as long as the medication serves a direct, legitimate purpose in a patient's care."

So the DEA regulation is a paper tiger. Its main function is to frighten physicians out of taking full advantage of Marinol. Fortunately, a few courageous doctors have persisted in prescribing Marinol for chronic pain, spasticity, migraine, depression, and other non-FDA-approved uses of THC.

MARINOL, MARIJUANA, AND DRUG TESTING

Marinol's legality has important implications for anyone who is subject to drug testing for employment, insurance, or law enforcement. So long as marijuana remains a Schedule 1 drug, you have no right to use it even medically, and you can be dismissed on the basis of a positive drug test. Since urine tests can detect marijuana metabolites in urine for one to five days after an occasional use, and up to six weeks for chronic users, this poses obvious problems for medical marijuana users.

One answer to this problem is to obtain a prescription for Marinol. Because Marinol is based on THC, it is indistinguishable from marijuana on the most commonly used drug screens. You have the right to test positive for any drug legally prescribed to you. Therefore, if you have a prescription for Marinol, you can't be disqualified for a marijuana-positive test!

There are, however, two limitations with this tactic. First, you will have to inform the medical review officer that you are taking Marinol, which involves disclosure of your medical condition. Second, new advances in drug detection technology have made it possible to distinguish marijuana from pure THC. According to Dr. Mahmoud El Sohly, director of the government's University of Mississippi marijuana research program, it is possible to detect certain non-THC cannabinoid metabolites that are present only in natural marijuana, not in Marinol, by using sophisticated gas chromatograph mass spectrometer (GCMS) analysis. You are unlikely to encounter such tests in the normal course of events. The standard practice is to test urine using immunoassay screens for THC metabolites, which are completely incapable of distinguishing between Marinol and marijuana. If, however, you arouse unusual suspicions, it is possible that you could be subjected to a more probing investigation by GCMS to determine whether you have used marijuana instead of Marinol.

3

MEDICINAL USES
OF MARIJUANA

DOONESBURY
by Garry Trudeau

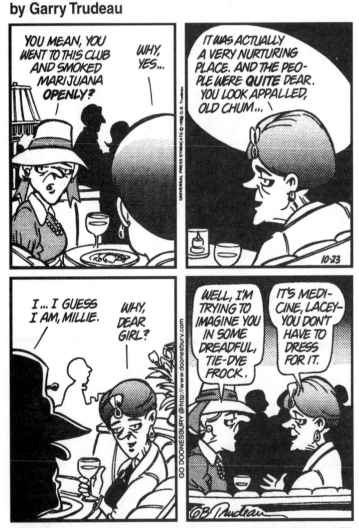

3

ANTIEMETIC AND APPETITE STIMULANT

The most familiar and best-established use of cannabis in modern medicine is as an antiemetic—that is, a treatment for severe nausea and vomiting—in connection with cancer nuclear medicine and chemotherapy.

Cannabis has been known to suppress nausea and stimulate appetite since its introduction to modern medicine in the nineteenth century. Recreational users have long been familiar with the "munchies," a heightened appetite (usually for snacking) that overtakes many users shortly after smoking.

Paradoxically, at extremely high doses, cannabis can actually precipitate nausea. Toxic reactions of this sort result from oral overdoses of the kind indulged in by the more adventurous hashish eaters.

The use of marijuana in cancer nuclear medicine and chemotherapy was documented in the early 1970s, when chemotherapy, like marijuana, was emerging into widespread popular use. Nuclear and chemotherapy drugs are by nature quite toxic, producing a nausea more profound than any associated with common diseases. Following their administration, patients can suffer hours of gut-wrenching vomiting, with "dry heaves" so severe as to result in broken bones. Nausea can persist for days or even weeks, leaving patients unable to eat. The distress can be so severe that some patients choose to forgo treatment altogether rather than endure it. A number of drugs are available by prescription for control of the side effects of nuclear medicine and chemotherapy, but they're not always satisfactory and can be extremely expensive.

Many patients find that a joint can relieve the misery of nuclear medicine and chemotherapy better than any other medicine. The remarkable value of marijuana was discovered serendipitously by young nuclear-medicine and chemotherapy patients familiar with its recreational use. Their stories came to the attention of doctors at Harvard University, among them Dr. Lester Grinspoon, whose own son Danny used it to treat himself during cancer chemotherapy. A flurry of research soon followed, in which both marijuana and oral THC were found to be effective in reducing nausea and vomiting from chemotherapy. Interest peaked in the early 1980s, when a number of states sponsored clinical research studies of medical marijuana.

In all, smoked marijuana was shown to be an effective antinauseant in six different state studies: New Mexico (250 patients), New York (199), California (98), Tennessee (27), Georgia (119), and Michigan (165).

In New Mexico, New York, and Tennessee, smoked marijuana proved to be effective in 90% of patients; in Georgia and Tennessee, it was effective in over 70%. In New Mexico and Tennessee, smoked marijuana also proved superior to oral THC. In Michigan, patients found smoked marijuana preferable to a conventional prescription antinauseant, Torecan.® In both New York and Tennessee, marijuana was effective for patients who had not been helped by THC.

The California study, which focused largely on oral THC, produced the least strong evidence for marijuana. Still, it found marijuana to be effective in 59% of patients, about the same as oral THC (57%). However, only 17% rated marijuana "highly effective," versus 30% for oral THC. About 11% of patients dropped out of treatment because of side effects, including anxiety, confusion, dizziness, depression, perceptual distortion, and so on. (Remarkably, "euphoria" was mentioned as a side effect, as if most cancer patients would not welcome some euphoria.)

The California study was conducted under protocols not calculated to yield good results. A participating researcher, oncologist Dr. Ivan Silverberg, noted, "The conditions were rigid, smoking times were prescribed; patients were not allowed to self-titrate their dose and were forced to smoke marijuana too quickly—and they could only smoke marijuana in a locked room. These restrictions seemed senseless to me. . . . To smoke marijuana under the conditions established in the California state program essentially placed the patient in a hostile environment."

The California state study was the only one to find oral THC superior to smoked marijuana. Apparently, most subjects chose to take capsules rather than smoke cigarettes out of an aversion to smoking. Many subjects had no prior smoking experience. Others complained about the harsh quality of the smoke from the government's marijuana. Researchers reported,

"The characteristics of the NIDA cigarettes may have been a factor in discouraging further use by experienced marijuana smokers. The cigarettes, even after proper storage, were dry and gave an acrid smoke. Their potency was noticeably low (1.2%–2.8%) at a time when street marijuana was increasing greatly in potency and availability."

Despite the promising findings about smoked marijuana in the state studies, official policy favored synthetic THC. In addition to being tainted by its illicit status, marijuana was criticized for being a natural plant whose ingredients and dosage were not rigorously controllable, whereas synthetic THC pills were regarded as more pharmaceutically pure and subject to precise regulation of dosage. In fact, as we have mentioned, the controllability of oral THC dosage was an illusion, given that subjects can much more readily adjust their own doses with smoked marijuana through self-titration. Still, the Reagan administration encouraged the use of oral THC rather than

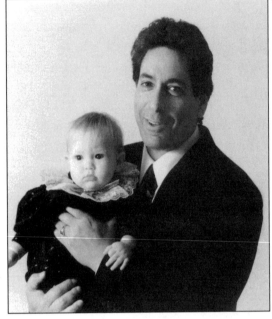

Steve Kubby, diagnosed at 28 with terminal cancer and given 2–3 years to live. Pictured celebrating his 50th birthday, with daughter Brook, age 9 months. He still tests positive for cancer but credits the use of marijuana to 22 years of a full and active life.

marijuana, and in 1986 the FDA approved it for cancer chemotherapy under the name of Marinol.

Still, many patients find that smoked marijuana works better than legal synthetic alternatives. One obvious advantage of marijuana is that many nuclear and chemotherapy patients are too sick to swallow a pill in the first place. Such patients find it much easier to inhale than to try to hold down a pill. In addition, of course, inhaled marijuana takes effect much faster, and its dosage is easier to control, making it less likely to produce unpleasant reactions.

Two other synthetic THC relatives, known as nabilone and levonantrodol, have been developed for cancer chemotherapy. Both are considerably less psychoactive than THC. Neither has won a large place in chemotherapy treatment, however.

More recently, in a pediatric study, a cannabinoid known as delta-8-THC was found to be completely effective in preventing vomiting in eight children who were cancer patients. Delta-8-THC is a close relative of delta-9-THC, with somewhat less psychoactive potency. Researchers observed "negligible" side effects in the children treated with delta-8-THC. Unfortunately, delta-8-THC is difficult to obtain, occurring only in trace quantities in natural marijuana as well as in Marinol, where it occurs as a byproduct of chemical synthesis.

Over the years, the market has become increasingly favorable to smoked cannabis as an antiemetic. While demand for Marinol has languished, thousands of cancer patients and physicians have turned to smoked marijuana—not that supplied by NIDA, of course, but good-quality, illicit grass. In some hospitals in San Francisco, the odor of marijuana wafts through the cancer wards, especially where there are large populations of younger, marijuana-familiar patients. The judgment of oncologists is that marijuana is a useful medicine. In a survey of oncologists by Mark Kleiman and Rick Doblin at Harvard University, nearly half of all respondents said they would prescribe natural cannabis if it were legal to do so. As the marijuana-experienced baby-boom generation ages, cannabis can be expected to become an ever more popular adjunct to cancer chemotherapy.

AIDS WASTING SYNDROME

An important new use of cannabis is in the treatment of nausea and appetite loss associated with AIDS. Many patients suffer severe weight and appetite loss, known as AIDS wasting syndrome, a condition whose impact on health and survival is severe. In Africa, wasting syndrome is a leading cause of death from AIDS.

Another cause of HIV-related appetite loss is AZT, the drug of choice for treating HIV infections. Unfortunately, AZT is also extremely nauseating. So is another popular AIDS drug,

Foscavira (foscarnet), used to treat an HIV-related eye infection, cytomegalovirus retinitis.

Many AIDS patients and doctors have found that marijuana helps them fight nausea and restimulate appetite and weight. The results can be dramatic: some people with aids (PWAs) have reported weight gains as great as 40 or 50 pounds in a few weeks. Marijuana has also been reported to be beneficial in relieving other HIV-related complaints, including leg cramps, headaches, neuropathy, and chronic fatigue.

The benefits of oral THC have been demonstrated in clinical testing of Marinol. An impressive 70% of HIV patients showed measurable weight gain after treatment with Marinol (Grinspoon, 91). One fifth of the patients had to discontinue treatment because of adverse side effects, which might have been lessened by the use of marijuana instead. In 1993, Marinol was approved by the FDA as safe and effective for treatment of AIDS-related wasting.

Unfortunately, the government has blocked similar research on marijuana. A study of marijuana and AIDS wasting syndrome by Dr. Donald Abrams of U.C. San Francisco was put on indefinite hold by the federal drug bureaucracy, which turned down his applications to obtain legal access to research marijuana. Even though Dr. Abrams's study protocol had been FDA-approved, the DEA refused to let him import cannabis from the Netherlands, and NIDA refused to let him use any of its own ample domestic supply.

Still, marijuana has become popular among AIDS patients and physicians, many of whom believe that it works better than Marinol. Cannabis has probably become the number one AIDS drug on the underground market. At the San Francisco Cannabis Cultivator's Club, AIDS patients account for some 80% of over 10,000 members.

One health concern connected with the use of marijuana for HIV patients is the risk of respiratory infections from smoking. Because of their compromised immune systems, PWAs are highly susceptible to the life-threatening lung infection pneumocystis carinii pneumonia (PCP). Smoking is known to lower resistance to respiratory infections. In a recent Johns Hopkins University study of drug-using PWAs, those who smoked illicit drugs, including marijuana and cocaine, were twice as likely to contract PCP. The implications of the study are not entirely clear, since almost all of the subjects also smoked cigarettes. Still, PWAs should approach smoking with caution.

One particular danger with smoked marijuana is contamination with bacteria and fungus spores, notably aspergillus fungus, which causes a lung disease that can be life-threatening to AIDS patients. Aspergillus infections have also been reported in cancer patients smoking marijuana for nausea. Patients should therefore take care not to smoke contaminated marijuana. See Chapter 5, "Using Marijuana as Medicine" for instructions on how to sterilize marijuana. Alternatively, many PWAs prefer to consume marijuana orally.

Opponents of medical marijuana have sometimes warned of the supposed immunosuppressive properties of THC as a potential problem for AIDS patients. The fact that the FDA has approved Marinol for treatment of AIDS should indicate that this claim is a red herring. As we have explained, the immunological effects of cannabinoids are disputed, but appear to have at most marginal effect, except perhaps for very heavy users or in certain exceptional cases. In any case, the particular immunosuppressive effects attributed to marijuana are not of a kind that should aggravate HIV infections. This is because the primary effect of HIV is to suppress the production of the immune system's T-cells, and there is no evidence that cannabinoids have any adverse impact on T-cell counts. In fact, one or two studies have suggested that marijuana may actually help boost T-cell counts. Other studies indicate that THC may modulate the immune system, stimulating certain responses in some instances and suppressing them in others.

Epidemiological surveys of recreational users have found no evidence that marijuana increases susceptibility to AIDS, as charged by some antidrug extremists. In fact, the recent San Francisco Men's Health Survey of 354 HIV-positive men actually found a decreased rate of progression to AIDS among marijuana users, although the difference was not statistically significant when adjusted for other factors, in particular the initial health of the different study populations.

OTHER ANTIEMETIC USES

Cannabis is useful not only for cancer chemotherapy, but also for other causes of nausea, vomiting, and appetite loss. These include various kinds of intestinal and kidney disease, adverse drug reactions, opiate addiction, and anorexia nervosa.

Some women use marijuana to treat morning sickness, despite obvious concerns about fetal exposure during pregnancy, especially during the first trimester. Though caution is always advisable in using drugs during pregnancy, marijuana doesn't appear to be as dangerous to fetal health as many other commonly used drugs, including tobacco, stimulants, and alcohol. Experts agree that marijuana does not cause gross birth defects. In any case, the risks of marijuana must be weighed against the benefits of relief from morning sickness, whose nausea can be so severe as to require hospitalization in some cases.

ANTICONVULSANT EFFECTS

One of the oldest established medicinal uses of cannabis is to treat epilepsy and muscle spasticity. Cannabis was used to treat epilepsy as far back as medieval Arabia and sixteenth-century Southeast Asia. When cannabis was first introduced to Western medicine, by Dr. William O'Shaughnessy in 1839, it was applied to treat convulsions caused by tetanus (lockjaw) and hydrophobia (rabies), and then puerperal convulsions, chorea, and strychnine poisoning (with varying success).

Since then, cannabis has been found useful for a host of spasm-inducing disorders, including multiple sclerosis, spinal injuries, dystonias, choreas, and many other conditions. Many of these diseases can be treated by a variety of prescription drugs, but not always satisfactorily, and often with debilitating, life-threatening, or otherwise intolerable side effects. Many patients report that they can reduce or eliminate their intake of toxic conventional medications and achieve better control of their complaints by smoking marijuana.

Though cannabinoids generally have anticonvulsant properties, they have also paradoxically been reported to precipitate muscle spasms in exceptional circumstances. As usual, this is most likely at higher doses. However, some animal studies have found that THC (though not CBD) at normal doses can excite nerve cell activity so as to promote convulsions. A few patients have been reported to exhibit myoclonic jerking or seizures after taking Marinol.

According to Dr. Paul Consroe of the University of Arizona, there is reason to think that CBD may have distinctive therapeutic value as an anticonvulsant. Not only does CBD appear to lack the stimulative activity of THC; it may also help counteract THC's muscle-exciting tendencies. For this reason, marijuana may be preferable to Marinol in treating muscle spasticity.

In normal subjects, marijuana also produces adverse effects on muscular coordination, a phenomenon familiar to anyone who has gotten too high. This deterioration, or ataxia, is most apparent in tasks that are complicated or require prolonged attention. One test is to try to hold your hand or finger steady in the middle of a slightly larger hole without touching the edges. These effects may to some extent counterbalance the benefits of cannabis for patients whose coordination is already impaired (for instance by multiple sclerosis).

EPILEPSY

Epilepsy, which occurs in numerous forms, is characterized by the misfiring of overactive brain cells, causing a seizure. Epileptic seizures can take the form of bodily convulsions (violent spasms), loss of consciousness, loss of coordination, altered sensory states, and, in extreme cases, coma or death. Epilepsy can arise from various causes, including accidents, disease, and genetic factors. Conventional treatments, which include a variety of prescription anticonvulsant drugs, benefit many patients, but 20% to 30% cannot be adequately controlled.

Many patients have found cannabis beneficial for two particular important kinds of epilepsy. The first of these is grand

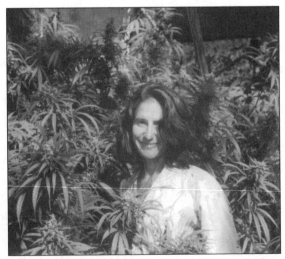

Valerie Corral founded the Wo-Men's Alliance for Marijuana after using marijuana to successfully control debilitating seizures which were the result of a car accident.

mal epilepsy, which is characterized by violent bodily spasms, caused by abnormal brain cell misfiring on both sides of the brain. Numerous grand mal epileptics report that they are able to completely eliminate seizures by smoking marijuana, sometimes in conjunction with their regular medication and sometimes without it.

Cannabis may also be useful for complex partial seizure disorders, which are associated with damage to the frontal or temporal lobes of the cerebral cortex. These disorders appear in various forms: a loss of consciousness, muscular twitching, and so on. In general, they are not easily treatable. Again, certain patients find cannabis can suppress these problems. In a study by Cunha, half of temporal focus partial epileptics obtained complete relief of seizures with CBD at doses some 10 times greater than the amount typically found in a joint; however, other studies have not been so promising.

Cannabis is by no means a cure-all for epilepsy. It is typically not useful for so-called petit mal or absence seizures; there is even evidence that CBD may counteract the efficacy of other drugs used for petit mal. Also, on at least one occasion, oral THC (at a dose of 20 mg) has precipitated a grand mal seizure in a patient with a previous history of epilepsy. Epileptics who are interested in trying cannabinoids should be careful about oral THC. Those who do use cannabinoids should be aware that they may become more susceptible to seizures when they withdraw from treatment.

MULTIPLE SCLEROSIS

Multiple sclerosis is a progressive, degenerative disease in which the brain and the spinal cord nerves are damaged by the gradual destruction of myelin, the protective tissue that coats them. Its symptoms include painful muscle spasms, numbness, impaired vision, loss of coordination and balance (ataxia), tremors, and weakness, progressing to incapacitation. There is no known effective treatment.

Many MS patients find that marijuana helps relieve their symptoms, particularly tremors and loss of coordination. One or two medical studies have been conducted with THC and marijuana. Though results were mixed, they did suggest that patients experience subjective benefits from both oral THC and marijuana. Remarkable benefits may occur in some instances, such as the case (reported by Dr. Lester Grinspoon) of Greg Paufler, who found that marijuana restored his ability to walk, run, speak, and engage in sex, all of which had been lost to MS. Likewise, Dr. Mikuriya reports successfully maintaining two MS patients with Marinol, supplemented by natural marijuana. One, a former aerospace engineer, suffered a relapse and became depressed and suicidal after losing his marijuana connection and being forced to rely on conventional therapies; he subsequently recovered after regaining access to cannabis.

There is some reason to think that cannabis may actually fight the progression of MS. This is because MS is a kind of autoimmune disease, caused by a hyperactive immune system. As we have seen, THC appears to have mild immunosuppressive effects. Though these effects don't seem to be important for most marijuana users, they may possibly benefit MS patients. This is suggested by recent research in which guinea pigs treated with THC resisted an MS-like infection known as experimental autoimmune encephalomyelitis. Untreated animals died. Autopsies showed reduced myelin inflammation in the THC-treated animals. There have been no human follow-up studies. However, as we shall see, there is reason to believe that THC is useful for other autoimmune diseases.

SPINAL CORD INJURIES, PARAPLEGIA, AND QUADRIPLEGIA

One of the most effective, yet underpublicized, uses of medical marijuana is for patients with spinal cord injuries. These patients often suffer severe chronic pain and muscle spasms, along with paralysis of the legs (paraplegia) or of both legs and arms (quadriplegia). Many find marijuana effectively relieves both spasticity and pain.

Spinal cord patients are commonly prescribed large doses of opiates, tranquilizers, and other debilitating and potentially dangerous drugs. Many find that they can dispense with these drugs altogether by using marijuana.

Although there have been no controlled studies of marijuana for spinal cord injuries, its usefulness is widely known both to patients and to physicians who specialize in pain control. In one survey, 22 out of 43 spinal cord injury patients were found to be using marijuana to control muscle spasms. Some VA hospitals allow marijuana to be smoked by paraplegics and quadriplegics in their wards.

OTHER MOVEMENT AND MUSCLE SPASM DISORDERS

Cannabis is helpful for numerous other movement disorders, some common and others too obscure to be listed here. (See accompanying table from Consroe and Sandyk, p. 65, 66, 69, and 70.) Because of the government's hostility to medical marijuana research, there have been virtually no human studies in this area. However, the uses described below have been confirmed by anecdotal reports.

MENSTRUAL CRAMPS AND LABOR PAIN

Many women find that marijuana relieves menstrual cramps or dysmenorrhea. This may result from the cannabinoids' suppression of prostaglandins. Dysmenorrhea was commonly treated with cannabis in the nineteenth century, and is said to have been the purpose for which Queen Victoria was prescribed cannabis by her personal physician. Unfortunately, of course, cramps are not the kind of "serious" disease for which physicians are likely to issue a triplicate Schedule 2 prescription, so women will probably have to wait for the arrival of over-the-counter cannabis before they can legally take full advantage of this comfort.

Cannabis has also traditionally been used to ease labor distress during childbirth. This is the single most ancient medical use of marijuana that is archaeologically confirmed. In a third-century tomb, Israeli archaeologists discovered the body of a girl who had apparently died in childbirth with traces of hashish at her bedside. Unfortunately, there has been absolutely no modern medical research on the efficacy of cannabis for childbirth.

INTESTINAL CRAMPS
Marijuana is sometimes useful for relieving abdominal cramps. In particular, patients have reported relief from colitis and Crohn's disease, two painful intestinal disorders that are thought to be related to nervous stress. Relief has also been reported from a rare genetic disease called Peutz-Jeghers syndrome, which causes similar bowel complaints. In the nineteenth century, cannabis was used to treat cholera, in order to relieve both diarrhea and vomiting. Today, of course, cholera can be successfully treated with other, modern therapies.

TOURETTE'S SYNDROME
This disorder is characterized by vocal and facial tics and jerking motions. Nervousness may be an aggravating factor. Some patients have reported relief by using marijuana.

DYSTONIAS

This class of disorders is characterized by involuntary muscular contractions, often creating a grotesque appearance. A five-patient study by Dr. Consroe showed some improvements from oral CBD.

BLACK WIDOW POISONING

The venom of the black widow spider causes severe, painful muscle cramps. A California herbalist (Carol Miller) says she found marijuana helpful in treating her husband for a black-widow bite. "His lower spine and upper body became wracked with horrible pain. The problem was getting him to smoke, because his jaw was locked up. A tincture would have worked better," she reports.

It is interesting that one of the earliest uses of cannabis in Western medicine was to treat lockjaw, or tetanus. Physicians reported mixed success with this treatment. Needless to say, anyone who comes down with tetanus, or has been bitten by a black widow, should seek immediate medical attention.

INTRAOCULAR PRESSURE REDUCER

GLAUCOMA

Glaucoma is a disease that causes excess fluid pressure in the eye (IOP—intraocular pressure). Over time, this pressure damages the optic nerve, causing permanent loss of sight and eventual blindness. [Some argue that other factors in addition to increased IOP must be present.] Some patients suffer painful, acute attacks with severe headaches and vomiting; in others, visual problems such as halos and blind spots are the most prominent symptoms. Glaucoma is the leading cause of blindness, affecting an estimated two million Americans over 35. It is normally treated by a variety of drugs and surgical procedures, but not always successfully.

It was discovered in the early 1970s that marijuana can help control glaucoma. At the time, it was widely believed that marijuana dilates the pupils of the eyes, a symptom that police hoped would help them uncover marijuana use. A UCLA research team, led by Drs. Robert Hepler and Thomas Ungerleider, tried to find out whether this was so. As part of their tests, they decided to give each subject a complete eye exam. As it turned out, marijuana did not dilate the eyes, but it did cause a significant reduction in IOP.

Follow-up studies confirmed that marijuana reduces IOP and can therefore help control glaucoma. Smoked marijuana and intravenously administered THC produced a consistent reduction in IOP, of about 20% to 40%, for a period of up to four hours. Studies showed that the effects were largely dose-independent, meaning that a heavier dose does not achieve further reduction of IOP. In many, if not all, cases, chronic use doesn't seem to result in tolerance; this implies that marijuana can be used for extended treatment.

Over the years, increasing numbers of patients have turned to marijuana for relief from glaucoma when other treatments have failed. Because marijuana is more psychoactive than other glaucoma treatments, it is generally used as a last resort. However, numerous patients say they have found relief from marijuana after other treatments have failed. Among them is Robert Randall, the first patient to obtain legal access to medical marijuana through the FDA. Randall, who had discovered that marijuana alone was able to prevent his sight from deteriorating, launched a lawsuit against the government after losing his home marijuana garden to a police raid. In 1978, he won a settlement in which the government agreed to supply NIDA-grown marijuana free of charge under a special compassionate IND FDA investigational drug protocol. Under the terms of this arrangement, Randall was technically considered to be a research subject in an FDA-approved single-person drug investigation, a process involving elaborate red tape and paperwork for Randall's physician. Difficult as it was for patients to qualify for this program, the compassionate IND protocol was expanded to some 30 patients until it was closed to new applicants by the Bush administration. Today, just eight patients still receive marijuana from the government, including Randall and one other glaucoma patient, Elvy Musikka.

Despite such well-documented precedents, the medical community has resisted endorsing marijuana for glaucoma. In his famous decision recommending that marijuana be rescheduled as a prescription drug, DEA judge Francis Young explicitly excluded glaucoma as an established use for cannabis, citing professional opposition from the American Academy of Ophthalmology, which claimed there was a lack of scientific evidence supporting marijuana's safety and efficacy.

One of the ophthalmologists' major concerns is that glaucoma patients need continual treatment to control their IOP. In Randall's case, this means smoking some 10 to 12 joints per day. Chain smoking of this kind poses obvious health concerns, especially respiratory hazards, over long periods of time. In addition, patients must spend all of their waking hours under the influence of THC; many subjects find this condition mentally incapacitating. Randall and others say they have developed a tolerance to the psychoactive effects of THC while staying sensitive to its therapeutic effects.

Marijuana is useful for wide-angle glaucoma, a condition that requires constant treatment. It does not control narrow or closed-angle glaucoma, a condition that manifests itself through acute, painful attacks. Although some patients find

that marijuana relieves the pain of these attacks, surgical treatment is essential to preserve vision.

For some mysterious reason, glaucoma doesn't respond well
to oral THC. Eye patients are virtually unanimous in claiming
that Marinol doesn't help them. Surprisingly, laboratory studies
have found that pure delta-9-THC does lower eye pressure
when administered intravenously. However, a trial of oral THC
capsules failed to produce results except at uncomfortably high
doses of 20 to 25 mg. Animal tests have shown that CBN and
delta-8-THC reduce IOP, but CBD does not. This is one of the
rare cases in which CBN has proven more medically effective
than CBD.

Many patients say that they find low-grade marijuana to be
as effective for treating glaucoma as high-potency sinsemilla.

Efforts have been made to develop topical eye drops that
would avoid the systemic psychoactive effects of THC. These
have been frustrated by the difficulty of formulating a solution
capable of delivering THC inside the eye. A topical cannabinoid
pharmaceutical was developed in the Caribbean, but it doesn't
seem to be available in the U.S. Recent studies suggest that a
form of anandamide prepared as eye drops might be useful.

The ocular action of THC is not entirely understood. THC
may reduce pressure by decreasing fluid secretion and/or
increasing fluid outflow from the eye. The latter effect may be
related to THC's well-known action of dilating the blood vessels in the eyes' conjunctiva. This produces the well-known
symptom of bloodshot eyes—a telltale, but unreliable, sign that
you've been smoking pot.

Another side effect of THC is to suppress tears. Dry eyes are
an annoying problem for some patients. Chronic dryness of the
eyes can lead to many other complications, such as cornea
ulceration, conjunctivitis, and keratitis. Some contact lens
users say they experience discomfort after smoking marijuana.

OTHER OCULAR EFFECTS

Marijuana is useful for eye diseases other than glaucoma. Erren has used marijuana to treat a drusen cyst, a growth that exerts pressure on his eyeball. Strangely, he says his condition responds to low-grade Mexican grass but not to high-potency sinsemilla. Once again, this indicates that marijuana's medical value depends on more than just THC, since low-grade Mexican marijuana often contains high percentages of CBD.

Cannabis may also be beneficial for eye disorders that are not related to ocular pressure. Many patients say marijuana helps relieve retinitis, an inflammation of the retina. One woman claims that marijuana helps her cope with optic nerve hypoplasia, a congenital underdevelopment of the eye that impairs her vision. She says marijuana helps her focus and see colors better, as well as reducing rapid abnormal eye movements. Other patients have reported that marijuana is useful for vision problems associated with macular degeneration, a progressive deterioration of the retina. Another patient reports that pot has helped him with amblyopic dyslexia, a difficulty with reading caused by blurry vision.

BRONCHODILATOR ASTHMA

Many patients find marijuana useful for relieving asthma attacks. Asthma is an allergic disorder in which the linings of the lungs become inflamed and swollen with phlegm, causing acute attacks of wheezing and breathlessness. Attacks are treated with bronchodilators, which relax and expand the air passageways of the lungs.

One of the proven effects of THC is to act as a bronchodilator. Studies have found that both smoked marijuana and oral THC can relieve asthmatic spasms. In comparison to standard bronchodilators, marijuana was found to have a milder peak effect, but to act longer. Aside from its psychoactivity, marijuana has fewer adverse side effects than other asthma drugs. The obvious drawback of inhaled marijuana is the smoke. Many asthmatics have a low tolerance for smoking of any kind. One answer is to use oral THC, but the difficulty is its long period of onset. At one point, Dr. Donald Tashkin of UCLA tested a THC spray inhaler for use with asthma. As it turned out, though, the THC droplets tended to be very irritating when they were inhaled. Other methods of inhaled delivery of pure THC have not been assessed.

Historically, marijuana was used to treat asthma in Mexican folk medicine. Introduced into the U.S. in the 1910s, this treatment was the first reported medical use of smoked marijuana.

ANALGESIC AND ANTI-INFLAMMATORY

Marijuana has been used to provide pain relief, or analgesia, for a wide variety of conditions, ranging from migraines and rheumatism to severe chronic pain caused by spine and nerve injuries, cancer, and other illnesses. Two thousand years ago, the Chinese used high doses of cannabis to prepare patients for major surgery. The analgesic properties of cannabis were exploited in the nineteenth century to treat migraines, rheumatism, menstrual pains, and terminal illness. These uses declined with the development of the more effective opiates, such as morphine, which were stronger and more consistent in their effects. However, many patients continue to find that cannabis is uniquely superior to prescription analgesics in controlling chronic pain.

Severe chronic pain is commonly treated with opioid narcotics (such as codeine or morphine) or with various synthetic analgesics. The opiates are notoriously addictive, and may become less effective as patients develop tolerance to them. In addition, many patients find themselves incapacitated by the stupefying and soporific effects of these drugs. Other, nonaddictive synthetic analgesics are available, but they are often not strong enough.

Many patients find that by smoking marijuana they can completely eliminate potent drugs such as opiate narcotics. A good example is Bill, who suffered sciatic pain in the back and legs following spinal fusion surgery: "My doctors prescribed heavy doses of prescription painkillers, including morphine and methadone, after my operation. My legal medicine left me feeling heavily drugged, yet still in pain and unable to lead a tolerable life. I became suicidal. Then one of my doctors suggested I try marijuana. When I tried it, I discovered that it relieved the excruciating, sharp, electric pain I had been experiencing. Although I still experienced some dull, throbbing pain, my level of discomfort was now tolerable, with no 'drugged' or negative side effects. Marijuana turned out to be a godsend for me." [Nevertheless, Bill was denied compassionate IND access to marijuana by the California Research Advisory Panel.]

According to the nineteenth-century authority, Dr. James B. Mattison, cannabis often turned out to be an "efficient substitute for the poppy" in the treatment of patients addicted to opium, chloral, or cocaine. "Its power, in this regard has sometimes surprised me," he reported.

The analgesic properties of cannabis are many, but are not well understood scientifically. The newly found cannabinoid receptor is thought to have analgesic functions that are activated by THC or THC analogs. It is not known whether THC acts entirely through the brain's higher, cognitive functions or also through some kind of action in the nerves. Both may be involved. Animals injected under the skin with very high doses of THC have shown reduced sensitivity to pain that was artificially induced by heat, pinching, chemical irritation, and so on; but the doses may be irrelevant to human use, and results have not been completely consistent. In a few cases, for example, THC has apparently caused heightened sensitivity to pain. Unlike THC, CBD by itself does not appear to be useful for treating pure pain. However, it may help alleviate pain indirectly by its sedative action or by relieving muscle spasms.

It's impossible to list all the painful diseases for which marijuana has been provided relief. Many are unusual diseases that do not respond to conventional medication, such as nail patellar syndrome (genetic underdevelopment of the nails or the kneecaps and other joints); spinal stenosis (squeezing of the spinal column); eosinophilia-myalgia syndrome (EMS—a disease caused by adulterated tryptophan); patellar chondromalacia (softening of the kneecaps); and pseudohypoparathyroidism (characterized by profuse growth of spurs on the bones). Many involve intense bodily pain associated with skeletal disorders or damaged nerves.

Marijuana is a favorite drug among disabled veterans with war injuries and is surreptitiously recommended at some VA clinics for hard-to-treat pain and muscle spasms. THC is said to be especially useful for "phantom pain" from amputated limbs; causalgias, or pain felt in limbs whose nerves have been damaged; and neuralgias, characterized by intense pain extending along the nerves—in particular, trigeminal neuralgia (tic douloureux), which causes acute stabbing pain in the jaw.

Cannabis has also been used with success to treat the chronic pain of advanced cancer. A study at the University of Iowa Clinical Research Center found that oral THC in doses of 5 to 10 mg was nearly as effective as 60 mg of codeine for relieving pain in 36 terminal cancer patients, with effects lasting several hours. At double doses, 20 mg THC was found to be even stronger than 120 mg of codeine; however, subjects found this dose too sedative and mentally incapacitating for their comfort. Of course, the psychoactive effects of THC depend greatly on the context in which it is taken, and they're much more pleasant to some people than to others. All but one of the patients in the Iowa study had no earlier marijuana experience; this made them more sensitive to adverse psychoactive effects.

For some, the psychoactive effect of cannabis may itself be analgesic. A final-stage cancer patient named Gordon used cannabis in a remarkable regimen of self-treatment for an advanced, terminal lymphoma that had spread to his pancreas and bone marrow. Gordon followed a rigorous regime of diet, exercise, and meditation, without any drugs except marijuana, which he used to aid his meditation. According to Gordon, pot did not make the pain go away, but helped him "learn to move right through it," reaching an ecstatic state of "vibrating blissfulness, where I felt very, very good." With repeated experiences, he found that the pain diminished and "the ability of the pain to grab my attention was lost."

Gordon, who cultivated his own marijuana, says that he was able to develop a specific strain that was especially effective in minimizing extreme pain. He found it was possible to hybridize different strains of cannabis that could specifically address different kinds of disorders, such as insomnia, physical and emotional disorders, and so on. Unfortunately, Gordon's labors were destroyed by the drug police.

MIGRAINE

Many patients report that marijuana is useful for treating migraine headaches. Migraine is a form of severe headache, often accompanied by nausea and vomiting, that lasts for hours and recurs chronically. Migraines are thought to be caused by the dilation of arteries in the brain. An estimated 20% of Americans, three quarters of them women, are afflicted by migraine.

During the nineteenth century, cannabis was considered to be the drug of choice for migraine. "Were its use limited to this alone, would be greater than most imagine," wrote Dr. J. B. Mattison in 1891. Today, patients are typically treated with aspirin, ergot derivatives, and a host of other medications, including opiates. As usual in medicine, these treatments do not always work. Many patients find that marijuana is more effective than conventional prescription drugs.

Unfortunately, little scientific research has been done on cannabis and migraine. There is some evidence that THC (but not CBD) inhibits the release of serotonin from blood platelet cells, a likely causal factor in migraines. Marijuana also seems to alter blood flow in the cerebrum, but the clinical implications of this fact for migraine are unclear. One investigator reported three cases in which former long-term pot smokers began having migraines shortly after giving up marijuana. Two had been free of migraines during their years of smoking; the third had had occasional headaches that pot quickly relieved. The author concluded that chronic marijuana use might suppress susceptibility to migraines.

Many patients report that they can avert a migraine attack by smoking a joint at the first warning of onset. Migraine attacks are often preceded by visual disturbances, weakness, dizziness, ringing in the ears, and other symptoms. If these symptoms are addressed promptly, full-blown migraine can be avoided. Patients say inhaled marijuana is preferable to oral preparations such as Marinol in such situations, because quick treatment is necessary. [There is no evidence that CBD or other non-THC cannabinoids are helpful against migraines.]

Paradoxically, on rare occasions, marijuana has also been reported to precipitate migraine attacks.

ARTHRITIS AND RHEUMATISM

Cannabis has often been used to treat rheumatism, arthritis, and related diseases. This was a classical use of cannabis in the nineteenth century, when it was said to be as effective as opium for severe rheumatism. Although it is no longer used much in modern orthodox medicine, many patients insist that it has unique benefits as a painkiller, antispasmodic, and anti-inflammatory agent.

Rheumatism includes various diseases marked by inflammation or degeneration of the joints, muscles, or connective tissue. Symptoms include pain, stiffness, loss of mobility, and inflammation of the joints. Severe cases can become completely debilitating. The first line of defense is typically aspirin for both pain and inflammation; severe cases often require stronger drugs, such as opiates for pain and corticosteroids for inflammation. These have dangerous side effects when they are taken regularly.

Many patients find cannabis helps relieve the chronic pain of severe arthritis, or rheumatism of the joints. In addition to its analgesic effects, cannabis can relieve the painful muscle spasms that often accompany rheumatic disease. David, who suffers fibromyalgia arthritis along with shingles (a painful disease caused by the chicken pox virus) and an injured leg, says marijuana "helps me to relax, dial into what's going on, break down the pain's control. . . . You can't make the pain go away," he says, "but you can learn to live with it."

In addition, marijuana may be useful as an anti-inflammant, reducing the swelling in arthritic joints. Animal studies have found that cannabinoids have anti-inflammatory properties. Chemically, this may be caused by an increase in the production of glucocorticoid hormones, which are used to treat inflammation, and a decrease in the synthesis of prostaglandin, a hormone involved in inflammation, which is also suppressed by aspirin. Experiments by E. A. Formukong of the University of London indicate that the nonpsychoactive cannabinoids cannabigerol (CBG) and CBD are more effective as anti-inflammants than THC. According to Dr. Mahmoud El Sohly, cannabichromene (CBC), a nonpsychoactive cannabinoid that has been found in high concentrations in certain strains of marijuana, particularly from South Africa, also has good anti-inflammatory effects. Surprisingly, anti-inflammatory properties have even been found in two noncannabinoid ingredients of marijuana, olivetol and cannflavin.

Other experiments have shown that THC can inhibit the aggregation of the immune system's platelet cells, which are a principal cause of inflammation. This may be one of THC's supposed "immunosuppressant" effects. Inflammation can be understood as the product of an overactive immune system, which attacks the body's own tissues. Many forms of rheumatism are thought to be essentially autoimmune in nature. In such cases, a degree of immunosuppression may well be beneficial.

A rheumatoid arthritis patient, Tom, who has studied the preparation of cannabis in cooking, says that marijuana helps relieve his inflammation when he took it in strong oral doses. He reports that oral ingestion is needed to achieve the desired effect because it is difficult to consume a sufficient dose through smoking. "It's much better eaten," says Tom. "Smoking gives muscle relaxation rather than pain relief." Tom's medical dose is 2 g, twice the standard recreational dose. Though this amount is likely to be incapacitating for normal daily functioning, Tom says he can take it at bedtime and wake up free of pain the next morning.

PSYCHOLOGICAL APPLICATIONS

Marijuana's psychoactive effects have been variously described as euphoriant (inducing a sense of good feelings and well-being), sedative (mildly tranquilizing), anxiolytic (anxiety-reducing), and hypnotic (sleep-inducing). Such mood-altering effects can be medically useful in treating depression and other affective disorders. At the same time, however, marijuana can have negative effects, including paranoia, irritability, dysphoria, depression, depersonalization, and amotivation. The interplay among these effects is complex and tricky, and their balance can alter from positive to negative in the same patient at various times. Because it is difficult for someone experiencing mood disorders to be objective, patients are strongly advised to consult a professional caregiver rather than to rely on self-medication for mood disorders.

Clinical Depression

Clinical depression is a serious illness, characterized by long-term, chronic, debilitating, sometimes suicidal feelings of sadness and low self-esteem. It should not be confused with simply feeling "down in the dumps," a state that is not properly treated with pharmaceuticals. Genuine clinical depression is regularly treated with a variety of prescription drugs: tricyclic antidepressants, monoamine oxidase (MAO) inhibitors, and, most recently, Prozac.® Bipolar depression, which is characterized by alternating high-energy "manic" and low-spirited "depressive" phases, is generally treated with lithium salts. Though most patients respond positively to prescription antidepressants, a minority do not, or cannot tolerate the side effects.

The mood-elevating properties of cannabis have been known since its first discovery as an intoxicant. The fabled Sufi credited with introducing hashish to Persia, Shaykh Haydar, is said to have made his monumental discovery after withdrawing into the fields in a state of depression. There he partook of the hemp plant, and "when he returned, his face radiated energy and joy, quite a contrast to his usual appearance as we knew him before." One of the first uses of cannabis in Western medicine, recommended by Dr. Jacques-Joseph Moreau de Tours, who spoke of the "mental joy" of hashish intoxication, was for treatment of depression and melancholia. Depression is also listed as treatable by cannabis in early twentieth-century medical texts. Modern clinical studies of depression have had more mixed results. In the late 1940s, one study with the artificial cannabinoid Synhexyl showed promising results, but was not confirmed in two follow-ups. Similarly disappointing results came from a 1973 study of eight depressed patients, in a double-blind test of THC versus a placebo. Not only did THC fail to relieve depression, but half of the patients experienced unpleasant anxiety and discomfort. However, the artificial set and setting of this experiment may not have been conducive to good results.

Still, physicians report that many patients who do not respond well to standard treatment find marijuana beneficial for depression. According to Dr. Mikuriya, who is a practicing psychiatrist, "the power of cannabis to fight depression is perhaps its most important property." Marijuana has been used successfully for both bipolar and regular clinical depression. Marinol has also been prescribed with success in such cases, despite DEA warnings against unlabeled uses.

Like most of marijuana's psychoactive effects, euphoria does not occur consistently in all patients. Anti-euphoric, or dysphoric, reactions have been observed in numerous studies, especially among older patients who are not accustomed to mood-altering drugs. Individual users may also experience differing effects, according to their own moods, expectations, and set and setting. When taken at the wrong time or in the wrong frame of mind, marijuana can provoke negative brooding.

In accordance with the perverse logic of DEA bureaucrats, euphoria has been listed as an "adverse reaction" of marijuana.

Of course, it's possible that some sullen or puritanical patients find euphoria disconcerting, but it's more likely that government prohibitionists are upset that others find happiness while breaking the law.

As noted by the medieval Arab/Persian author of the Mukzun-ul-Udwieh, hemp drugs can have contrary stimulant and sedative effects: "They at first exhilarate the spirits, cause cheerfulness, excite the imagination into the most rapturous ideas, produce thirst, increase appetite, excite concupiscence. Afterward the sedative effects begin to preside, the spirits sink, the vision darkens and weakens; and madness, melancholy, fearfulness, dropsy, and such like distempers are the sequel."

Anti-Anxiety Agent

Cannabis is often said to have calming and anxiety-reducing effects. Medically, it is used for many of the same problems as minor tranquilizers such as the benzodiazepines Librium® and Valium,® including convulsive-movement disorders, chronic pain, and so on. Many patients feel that cannabis is superior to the benzodiazepines and other sedatives because it produces less dulling of mental acuity.

However, contrary to the popular image of marijuana as producing a "laid-back" state, it can also aggravate anxiety. This can be seen in the well-known phenomenon of "panic reactions," which often trouble inexperienced users, especially at high levels of THC. Although panic reactions quickly fade with the effects of the drug, they can be frightening enough for some users that they seek medical help. In milder cases, users may simply be discomfited by heightened paranoia, self-consciousness, and anxiety. Panic reactions are sufficiently common that they have been mentioned in medical studies as a major impediment to medical use of cannabis. One aggravating factor here, as we have mentioned, is that the set and setting of medical studies tend to inspire nervousness rather than relaxation.

Experienced marijuana users appear to be less prone to panic attacks than inexperienced users. [Of course, one reason for this could be that persons who suffer panic reactions are less inclined to become regular users in the first place.] A study of 17 subjects by Mathew and Wilson, at Duke University, found that marijuana smoking increased anxiety in inexperienced users, but decreased it in experienced ones. Inexperienced users also reported increased depression. The authors related this to differences in cerebral blood flow in the two groups; unlike the experienced users, inexperienced users appeared to suffer a decrease in blood flow in the brain, perhaps caused by anxiety.

Other evidence suggests that the anxiety-enhancing effects of marijuana result mainly from THC and can be counteracted by CBD. Animal studies have generally found CBD to have anxiolytic and antipsychotic effects. A study by A. W. Zuardi found that eight subjects given pure THC consistently felt more "discontented," "withdrawn," "troubled," "muzzy," "incompetent," "feeble," and "drowsy." When given CBD, they were apt to feel more "alert," "quick-witted," "clear-minded," "tranquil," and "gregarious." The combination of THC and CBD yielded intermediate effects. All this indicates that marijuana with CBD is preferable to Marinol for dealing with anxiety. Because of its ambivalent effects, few physicians recommend cannabis specifically for anxiety in the absence of other problems such as pain or muscle spasms. However, for the latter disorders, cannabis may be a good substitute for prescription tranquilizers.

Obviously, considerable caution must be used in recommending marijuana to patients with serious mental disturbances. Some studies have found that cannabis is associated with a higher incidence of schizophrenia. Though there is no evidence that cannabis actually precipitates schizophrenia, it may well make preexisting problems worse.

On the other hand, there is evidence that recreational use of cannabis may have a sedative effect on many mental patients. A recent survey of 79 psychotics found that those who used marijuana recreationally tended to report less anxiety, depression, insomnia, and physical discomfort. Relatively few experienced adverse effects such as paranoia and hallucinations. In contrast, most patients who drank alcohol reported that it aggravated their problems. The authors concluded that marijuana may have a "useful, calming effect" in some patients.

Cannabis has also been used for patients with senile dementia or Alzheimer's disease, to relieve anxiety, hostility, insomnia, and anorexia. A recent Unimed study found that Marinol helped reduce both depression and anorexia in Alzheimer's patients.

Another anecdotal use of marijuana is for chronic fatigue syndrome (CFS), a mysterious illness of unknown etiology. Symptoms of CFS include debilitating fatigue, headaches, depression, muscle weakness, and other symptoms. Many CFS patients state that marijuana makes them feel better. Unfortunately, there have been no medical studies of this treatment.

Some enthusiasts claim to use marijuana for "stress." However, this is not a recognized medical indication for mood-altering drugs. Stress is not an internal mental disorder, but rather the effect of external pressures from everyday life. In contrast, tranquilizers are generally reserved for what are called "severe anxiety disorders," involving an inherent constitutional problem. Mood-altering drugs are not medically recommended as a way of coping with reality; on the contrary, such use is generally condemned by orthodox medicine. A widely deplored evil of cannabis abuse is its ability to encourage escapism and discourage users from dealing with their problems. This can be seen in the so-called amotivational syndrome, a tendency for users to disengage from the real world. "Stress reduction" may therefore be less a legitimate medical use for marijuana than an excuse for recreational escapism.

INSOMNIA

Many patients find that marijuana helps them sleep better. In the nineteenth century, cannabis was widely recognized as an effective hypnotic; Dr. J. R. Reynolds strongly recommended it for "senile insomnia." Tales of early hashish explorers are filled with accounts of dreams, torpor, and immobility, aggravated no doubt by heavy doses. In fact, overdoses of cannabis are known to make people pass out.

The hypnotic properties of cannabis are of special value to chronic pain patients, many of whom rely on it for a good night's sleep. Quite a few healthy people also take a toke or two every night before bedtime to help them get to sleep. Medical studies have found that both THC and CBD by themselves help improve sleep.

Like other effects of marijuana, sleepiness is not a consistent effect. In fact, many users find that marijuana keeps them awake. In general, as we have mentioned, cannabis tends to be most exciting in the first hour or so after smoking, then gradually becomes more sedative.

In some instances, marijuana may suppress dreaming. Studies of sleeping subjects have shown that THC tends to suppress rapid-eye-movement (REM) sleep, during which dreams occur. These effects are most apparent at very high doses, and may decline with chronic use. However, one Freudian psychotherapist complains that her pot-smoking patients don't have enough dreams to report.

Former heavy users sometimes report insomnia and vivid dreams after giving up marijuana. These are withdrawal effects; they subside after a few weeks.

ALCOHOLISM AND DRUG DEPENDENCY

Cannabis may provide a safer substitute for other, more harmful drugs, both recreational and medical. As we have seen, many patients find that marijuana can eliminate their dependence on potent prescription drugs, such as opiates, antidepressants, anti-inflammants, and so on, many of which have dangerous side effects when used regularly.

In addition, many ex-alcoholics and other ex-drug addicts say they have been able to kick their habits by using marijuana as a substitute. Because marijuana is less toxic and debilitating than heavy alcohol or hard-drug abuse, this is typically a healthy development. Unlike marijuana, excessive alcohol can be toxic to the liver, the brain, and the digestive and circulatory systems. Like opiates, alcohol can also be physically addicting, producing life-threatening withdrawal symptoms in some cases.

Many alcoholics say that they have reestablished control of their lives by giving up alcohol for marijuana. Benefits include avoidance of binge-drinking blackouts and hangovers, reduced depression, improved eating habits, and reduced hostility and violence toward others. A few ex-junkies report similar benefits from marijuana as a replacement for opiates. Marijuana has sometimes been proposed as a treatment for addiction withdrawal symptoms. There is some evidence that THC can reduce the effects of opiate withdrawal. Animal studies have shown that THC reduces opiate withdrawal in dependent rodents. In the nineteenth century, cannabis was tried in the treatment of delirium tremens, the shaking and convulsions associated with alcohol withdrawal; however, the results were not especially good. In general, marijuana appears to be less useful for withdrawal than as an outright replacement for recreational use of other drugs.

Tobacco addicts have sometimes been known to substitute marijuana for cigarettes. The benefits of substitution are more doubtful in this case. Puff for puff, marijuana smoke is every bit as harmful to the lungs as tobacco—in addition to which, of course, it is more psychoactive and more expensive. However, some nicotine addicts have successfully used marijuana to wean themselves from cigarettes. The joint provides oral satisfaction and the act of inhalation may also have a placebo effect. Once the nicotine addiction ends, smokers can taper off the marijuana.

Cannabis substitution is by no means well accepted by the drug treatment establishment, which in recent years has become largely devoted to the goal of total drug abstinence, as preached in the twelve-step recovery programs such as Alcoholics Anonymous. However, twelve-step programs don't work for everyone.

In the 1970s, marijuana was investigated as a possible aid in alcohol treatment programs, but the results were disappointing. It had been suggested that recreational use of marijuana might help stem alcoholism, on the assumption that users tended to substitute one for the other. Unfortunately, subsequent studies found heavy combination use of marijuana with alcohol and drugs: some 50% of all marijuana users are also heavy drinkers. In fact, many users report that pot smoking makes them drink more, because it makes them thirsty.

Still, there is some evidence that marijuana may indeed stem alcohol and other drug abuse. According to Vera Rubin, who studied ganja use in Jamaica, alcoholism accounted for only 1% of mental hospital admissions there, as compared to 55% on the nearby island of Barbados, where ganja use is uncommon. In the Netherlands, health officials believe that the legal availability of cannabis has helped reduce the abuse of harder drugs. Recent studies by the RAND Corporation found that teen marijuana use tends to increase with decreasing access to alcohol, and that states with higher marijuana use have fewer emergency-room visits for drug abuse. Another study, by Frank Chaloupka of the University of Illinois at Chicago, found that states with liberal marijuana laws tend to have fewer auto accidents than other states, perhaps because they have less drunken driving.

Table 1
Reported Effects of Marijuana Treatment on Features of Neurological Disorders Described in the 19th Century and Possible Contemporary Analogies to These Neurological Disorders

Disorders of the 19th century	Contemporary disorders	Effect of marijuana
Convulsions: recurrent, general, tonic, clonic	Tonic-clonic seizures generalized epilepsy	Benefit
Convulsions, petit mal	Absence seizures, generalized epilepsy	No effect
Spasms of torticollis and writer's cramp	Dystonic movements; spasmodic torticollis; writer's cramp	No effect
Rheumatic chorea generalized chorea	Choreic movements; Sydenham's chorea; Huntington's chorea	Benefit, no effect
Tremor of paralysis agitans	Resting tremor; Parkinson's disease	No effect
Tonic painful spasms; jerky movements of spinal sclerosis	Spasticity and ataxia; spinal cord injury; multiple sclerosis	Benefit, no effect
Pain of neuropathy, e.g., sciatica	Sustained pain; neuropathic pain	No effect
Pain of neuropathy, e.g., trigeminal neuralgia	Paroxysmal pain; neuropathic pain	Benefit
Migraine headache	Migraine headache	Benefit

© Dr. Consroe and Dr. Sandyk, CRC PRESS

OTHER AUTOIMMUNE INFLAMMATORY DISEASES

Cannabis may be useful in treating many other diseases characterized by inflammatory and autoimmune disorders. One example is multiple sclerosis, which is a kind of immune attack against the nerve cells' protective myelin coating. Experiments

Table 2
Predicted Effects of (—)–Δ^9–Tetrahydrocannabinol (THC) and Cannabidiol (CBD) on Contemporary Neurological Disorders Based on Their Reported Activity in Animal Models

Disorder or symptom	Animal model	Drug	Predicted effect
Partial (simple and complex) seizures	Focal seizures	THC	Aggravate or benefit
		CBD	Benefit
Tonic-clonic seizures (grand mal)	Maximal generalized seizures	THC	Benefit
		CBD	Benefit
Absence seizures (petit mal)	Minimal generalized seizures	THC	No effect or aggravate
		CBD	No effect
Dystonia, Huntington's chorea, Tourette's syndrome, and tardive dyskinesia	Reserpine-induced hypokinesia	THC	Benefit
		CBD	Benefit
Parkisonism: hypokinesia	Reserpine-induced hypokinesia	THC	Aggravate
		CBD	Aggravate
Dystonia	Inherited dystonia	CBD	Benefit
Huntington's chorea	L-Pyroglutamate-induced behavioral disturbance	CBD	Benefit
Spasticity	Polysynaptic and monosynaptic reflexes	THC	Benefit, or aggravate
		CBD	Benefit
Cerebellar ataxia	Cannabinoid-induced ataxia	THC	Aggravate
		CBD	No effect
Migraine headache	Nociception, edema and prostaglandins	THC	Benefit
		CBD	No effect

have shown that THC can reduce myelin inflammation in animals with MS-like disorders.

Patients have reported benefits for a host of other painfully debilitating, chronic autoimmune/inflammatory disorders, many of them obscure. None of these applications has yet been investigated in controlled human studies. However, based on interviews with over 200 Cannabis Buyers' Club patients and 30 years of private practice, Dr. Tod Mikuriya has observed that "cannabis appears to be a unique immunomodulator analgesic," useful in a wide variety of conditions, including the following:

MUSCULOSKELETAL
Post-traumatic arthritis, rheumatoid arthritis, osteoarthritis, nail-patellar-tooth disease, melorheostosis, osteochondrosis, spinal stenosis, EMS (eosinophilia-myalgia syndrome), patellar chondromalacia.

CENTRAL AND PERIPHERAL NERVOUS SYSTEM
Seizure disorders; degenerative diseases of the central and peripheral nervous systems, including cerebral palsy, multiple sclerosis, Charcot-Marie-Tooth disease, post-viral encephalopathy and neuropathy; tic douloureux; diabetic neuropathy; post-injury CNS or PNS pain; glaucoma; drusen of the optic nerve; oculomotor post-congenital spastic blindness; migraine headache.

GASTROINTESTINAL SYSTEM
Gastritis, duodenal ulcer, regional enteritis, Crohn's disease, colitis (spastic and ulcerative), hepatitis, Peutz-Jeghers disease.

GENITOURINARY
Cystitis, dysmennorhea, orchitis, epididymitis.

ENDOCRINE
Thyroidtis, amyloidosis, scleroderma, lupus, premenstrual syndrome, pseudohypoparathyroidism.

SKIN
Intractable itching.

EAR, NOSE, AND THROAT
Meniere's disease, motion sickness, sinusitis, allergic rhinitis.

CARDIOPULMONARY
Asthma, chronic cough.

ANTIBIOTIC

There is some evidence that cannabis has antibacterial properties. Researchers in Czechoslovakia have found that extracts containing cannabidiolic acid can suppress certain bacteria, including certain antibiotic-resistant staphylococci. Applications of cannabis extract have relieved pain and infection from cuts and burns.

Some people also use topical cannabis solutions to treat viral infections such as herpes and corns. So far, such reports are strictly anecdotal. Further research is needed to determine whether cannabis truly has antimicrobial value.

ANTI-TUMORAL

It is sometimes claimed that marijuana has anti-tumoral properties. Experiments with laboratory animals have shown that injections of THC, CBN, and other cannabinoids can reduce the size of cancers. However, there have been no human studies of these effects.

DISPUTED USES

CHOREAS
This category of disorders is characterized by ceaseless, rapid, complex, jerky movements. In the nineteenth century,

cannabis was used to treat Sydenham's chorea, a children's illness caused by rheumatic fever, which is now quite rare. More common today is Huntington's chorea, a progressive, degenerative disease of genetic origin, which claimed folk singer Woody Guthrie. Trials with CBD have shown mixed results.

Table 3
Reported Effects of Marijuana (MJ), (—)-Δ⁹-Tetrahydrocannabinol (THC) and Cannabidiol (CBD) on Contemporary Neurological Disorders

Disorder	Major symptom	Drug	Effect
Focal epilepsy	Partial (simple and complex) seizures	MJ CBD	Benefit Benefit or no effect
Generalized epilepsy	Tonic-clonic seizures (grand mal)	MJ THC Analog CBD	Benefit Benefit Benefit or no effect
Generalized epilepsy	Absence seizures (petit mal)		
Dystonias	Dystonia	CBD	Benefit
Huntington's disease	Chorea	CBD	No effect
Tourette's syndrome	Tics	MJ	Benefit
Tardive dyskinesia	Oro-buccal-lingual dyskinesia	MJ	No effect
Parkinson's disease	Resting tremor; rigidity hypokinesia	MJ CBD	No effect Aggravate
Multiple sclerosis and spinal cord injury	Spasticity; intention tremor; ataxia	MJ THC	Benefit Benefit
Neuropathic conditions	Sustained pain	CBD	No effect
Migraine	Pain and other symptoms	MJ	Benefit

Table 4
Therapeutic Potential of Marijuana (MJ), (—)–Δ⁹–Tetrahydro-cannabinol (THC) and Cannabidiol (CBD) on Contemporary Neurological Disorders

Disorder	Major symptom	Drug	Therapeutic Effect
Focal epilepsy	Partial (simple and complex) seizures	MJ	+
		THC	-/+
		CBD	+/-
Generalized epilepsy	Tonic-clonic seizures (grand mal)	MJ	+
		THC	+
		CBD	+/
Generalized epilepsy	Absence seizures (petit mal)	MJ	/+
		THC	-/+
		CBD	-/+
Dystonias	Dystonia	MJ	+/-
		THC	+/-
		CBD	+
Huntington's disease	Chorea	MJ	+/-
		THC	+/-
		CBD	--
Tourette's syndrome	Tics	MJ	+
		THC	+/-
		CBD	+/-
Tardive dyskinesia	Oro-buccal-lingual dyskinesia	MJ	-
		THC	+/-
		CBD	+/-
Parkinson's disease	Resting tremor; rigidity hypokinesia	MJ	-
		THC	-/+
		CBD	-
Multiple sclerosis and spinal cord injury	Spasticity; intention tremor; ataxia	MJ	+
		THC	++
		CBD	+/-
Neuropathic conditions	Sustained pain	MJ	-/+
		THC	
		CBD	--
Neuropathic conditions	Paroxysmal pain	MJ	+/-
		THC	
		CBD	
Migraine	Pain and other symptoms	MJ	+/-
		THC	
		CBD	-/+

Therapeutic potential is rated from +++ to ---; ratings indicate excellent (+++), good (++), and fair (+) evidence for efficacy; equivocal or uncertain evidence for (+/-) or against (-/+) efficacy; and fair (-), good (--), and excellent (---) evidence for lack of efficacy. A blank space indicates no data or reports.

TARDIVE DYSKINESIA
This disorder, which manifests itself in involuntary chewing and darting of the tongue, is an insidious side effect of the long-term use of antipsychotic drugs. Contrary to expectations, marijuana has yet to show evidence of clinical efficacy. On the other hand, it does not cause TD, as some critics have alleged.

As always, cannabis should be approached cautiously by people with psychotic disorders, since it can aggravate (as well as alleviate) such illnesses.

PARKINSONISM
Parkinson's disease is a degenerative, progressive disorder, characterized by slow movement (hypokinesia), stiffness, and tremor. Some patients say marijuana helps alleviate Parkinsonism. However, others say it aggravates hypokinesia. Clinical studies have been disappointing. Contrary to some claims, there is no reason to think that cannabis causes Parkinsonism.

CEREBRAL PALSY
Some say that cannabis is helpful for cerebral palsy, a movement disorder caused by central nervous system injury during birth. There have been no studies of this application.

NON-USES
Disorders for which marijuana doesn't seem to work include writer's cramp; cramps, sprains, and muscle strains caused by physical stress or injury; simple muscle pains; and stomachaches.

4

THE MEDICAL
EFFECTS OF MARIJUANA

DOONESBURY
by Garry Trudeau

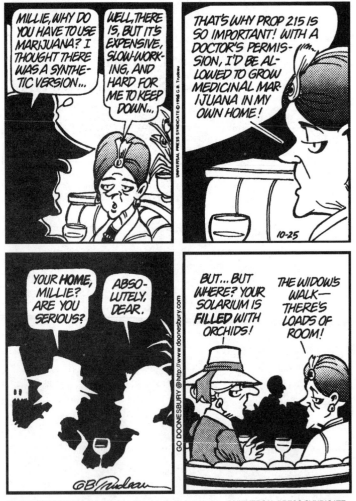

4

HEARTBEAT AND BLOOD PRESSURE

Right after smoking, THC speeds up the heart by about 30 to 60 beats per minute. This lasts for the first hour or so. There is no reason to think it is dangerous, any more than the fast heartbeat caused by jogging or by a game of tennis. However, it may be a problem if you have heart disease. Some heart patients experience chest pains or other circulatory discomfort when they smoke marijuana. Of course, heart patients should consult their doctors and before using it.

Frequent users develop some tolerance to tachycardia (fast heartbeat). Tachycardia can be blocked by the prescription drugs known as beta blockers, such as propranolol, which is sometimes prescribed for high blood pressure and other circulatory ailments. If you're concerned about tachycardia, then, you might find it useful to ask your doctor for a beta blocker prescription if you're thinking of using marijuana.

Tachycardia may also be aggravated when THC is combined with nortriptyline, a common antidepressant.

THC may affect blood pressure, but not in such a clear-cut and consistent way. Over a short time, along with the tachycardia, THC may cause a small increase in blood pressure. However, this doesn't happen for everyone. Chronic use may also cause a small decrease in blood pressure.

Marijuana's effects on blood pressure depend not only on dosage, but also on posture. THC tends to increase blood pressure when you're lying down and decrease it when you're standing up. This can cause momentary dizziness, or even a fainting spell, when you stand up suddenly, because blood rushes out of your brain. Some heavily dosed marijuana users have been known to pass out on the floor.

If you feel dizzy or faint, sit or lie down so that you don't fall. After a few minutes the sensation will disappear. Most people who have experienced unpleasantness from marijuana just let the symptoms fade away, usually in a matter of minutes or, more rarely, hours.

Because THC has unpredictable effects on blood pressure, experts disagree as to whether it's helpful or harmful for treating high blood pressure, or hypertension. Some hypertensive patients say marijuana helps them control their blood pressure, but this hasn't been checked in scientific studies.

In its report, *Marijuana and Health* (82), the National Academy of Sciences warned:

> The smoking of marijuana causes changes in the heart and circulation that are characteristic of stress. But there is no evidence that it exerts a permanently deleterious effect on the normal cerebrovascular system.

The situation is quite different for a user with an abnormal heart. There is much evidence that marijuana increases the work of the heart. This increase in the workload is dangerous for patients with hypertension, cerebrovascular disease, and coronary atherosclerosis.

Confusingly, the American Glaucoma Society expressed the opposite concern:

> From the standpoint of glaucoma management . . . the most disturbing adverse reaction is systemic hypotension (low blood pressure), which has been observed with the use of oral and intravenous cannabinoids as well as marijuana inhalation.

Given these conflicting views, the best advice for a heart patient is to talk to your doctor and watch the effects of marijuana on your own heart rate and blood pressure.

PREGNANCY

In general, women should completely avoid drugs during pregnancy. This rule applies to marijuana along with all other drugs. However, marijuana isn't so dangerous to fetal health that it can't be used medically when it's necessary.

Marijuana has not been shown to cause gross birth defects. Recent studies have dispelled concerns, widely publicized by anti-pot propagandists, that marijuana causes fetal alcohol syndrome. Some researchers believe that marijuana may result in slightly reduced birth weight, which is considered a problem for infant health. However, one study found that marijuana may increase birth weight instead. Other researchers say that regular maternal marijuana use may slightly retard later development. Here again, though, the evidence is mixed: a study of Jamaican women found improved development scores in children born to ganja-smoking mothers.

The therapeutic benefits of medical marijuana must be weighed against these hypothetical risks. Obviously, if the mother has a life-threatening disease such as cancer, it doesn't make much sense to worry about the slight risk of fetal harm from marijuana. Again, if a woman finds marijuana helpful for morning sickness, the risks to the fetus can very well be worse if the nausea isn't treated.

MYTHOLOGICAL DANGERS

Many other adverse effects have been attributed to marijuana by anti-pot propagandists (indeed, claims of marijuana's toxicity, once they're made, never die). Among them are impaired fertility and reproduction, harm to the immune system, brain damage, chromosome and cell damage, and birth defects. These charges, which were widely publicized in the 1980s by the government and by anti-pot groups such as PRIDE and the Partnership for a Drug-Free America, are inaccurate.

REPRODUCTION

Experts for the National Institute on Drug Abuse now say that pot has no permanent effect on the male or female reproductive system. Not a single case of impaired fertility has ever been found among marijuana users of either sex. At most, it's possible that marijuana may cause mild, temporary disruptions in ovulation, fertility, and menstrual cycles. Research has also failed to confirm claims that marijuana lowers testosterone and other sex hormones in men or women.

BRAIN DAMAGE

NIDA experts have also admitted that pot doesn't kill brain cells. This myth was based on some highly questionable animal experiments, by Dr. R. G. Heath, in which monkeys were exposed to uncertain levels of smoke. It has been disproven by careful research at the National Center for Toxicological Research and SRI International. Human studies in Jamaica and Costa Rica have found little evidence of cognitive defects even after long-term, very heavy marijuana use.

CHROMOSOME AND CELL DAMAGE

Charges that THC causes chromosome and gene damage are based on outdated studies of the 1970s that have now been conclusively discredited.

IMMUNE SYSTEM

Pot critics often charge that THC impairs the immune system. Supposed immunosuppressive effects of THC were first reported in laboratory studies of the 1970s, which found that it mildly inhibited the activity of certain immune cells, chiefly T-lymphocytes. Not a single case of human immune suppression due to THC has been observed epidemiologically or in clinical studies. If human immunosuppressive effects do occur, they're reversible, subtle, and of very little relevance to most users.

Cannabinoids do influence the immune system, by interacting with a special chemical receptor in immune-system cells. There's no reason to assume that this is harmful, since the action of THC on the immune system is complex and subtle. Recent animal studies suggest that THC may actually stimulate immune cells in some situations, so cannabinoids might more accurately be considered to be immune system modulators than suppressants.

Some individuals may be particularly susceptible to adverse immune effects. In one case, a patient had genital warts (papilloma virus infection) that resisted treatment whenever he used marijuana. Other lab studies have shown that marijuana may promote herpes infections in animals. But on the other hand, some patients insist that marijuana relieves herpes. As always, it's best for patients to be alert for any reactions, both adverse and beneficial.

Unlike oral THC, smoked marijuana impairs the immune response of the lungs. This is not because of the cannabinoids, but because of pyrolytic toxins in the smoke, which attack the lung's immune cells, its hairlike cilia, and other defense mechanisms. These hazards can be avoided by taking marijuana orally, or by various smoke reduction techniques described below.

VIOLENCE

Contrary to myth, marijuana does not promote violent behavior. In fact, it tends to suppress it. When marijuana first became a public concern in the 1920s, its opponents spread scare stories about reefer-crazed Mexicans driven to murder and mayhem. Subsequent scientific studies found exactly the opposite effect.

According to the National Academy of Sciences, "Both ret-rospective and experimental studies in human beings have failed to yield evidence that marijuana use leads to increased aggression. Most of these studies suggest quite the contrary effect. Marijuana appears to have a sedative effect, and it may reduce somewhat the intensity of angry feelings and probability of interpersonal aggressive behavior."

The laid-back hippie, not the murderous bandido, turns out to be the more realistic stereotype of the pot smoker.

MOTIVATION

Marijuana has been said to cause an "amotivational syndrome," characterized by a loss of ambition, motivation, and interest. The evidence for this is disputed. Believers cite examples of adolescents who have suddenly lost interest in school, friends, and so on after starting to smoke pot. Skeptics counter that marijuana doesn't induce amotivation, but that persons who already have motivational problems may be attracted to heavy marijuana use. They note that many highly motivated, success-ful professionals are pot smokers.

In fact, marijuana does have sedative, relaxing properties. Animal studies have shown that monkeys are less likely to strain for a banana after being given marijuana. [Of course, the monkeys may realize there's no point in knocking themselves out for a lab experiment!] This may explain the "laid-back" stereotype of human potheads. However, it doesn't show that marijuana robs adults of their careers, families, or goals. If you already have a clear sense of goals, marijuana won't "demoti-vate" you.

LONG-TERM HEALTH CONCERNS

Though marijuana is extremely safe with moderate use, the likelihood of adverse effects naturally rises with long-term, heavy use. Because of the relative novelty of marijuana in developed countries, epidemiological evidence of its long-term effects is still scarce. Studies of long-term users in Jamaica, Costa Rica, and Greece have found surprisingly little evidence of physiological problems even with extremely heavy use (10 or more joints per day), although they did detect subtle cognitive and psychological defects.

It wasn't till 1993 that a controlled study produced actual epidemiological statistics on the long-term safety of marijuana for users who don't smoke tobacco. The study, conducted by the Kaiser Permanente Center for Health Research, compared the health records of 452 non-tobacco-smoking daily marijuana users with those of 450 non-users ("Health Care Use by Frequent Marijuana Smokers Who Do Not Smoke Tobacco," *West J Med* 1993: 158). It found that the marijuana smokers had a 19% greater risk of respiratory diseases than non-users, confirming the suspicion that marijuana smoking causes lung disease in a way much like that of cigarettes.

The study also found that the daily marijuana smokers had a 30% higher risk of injuries than non-users, suggesting a higher incidence of accidents caused by intoxication. Oddly, the injury risks were highest for long-term daily marijuana users (15 years or more), but were not significantly higher for newer users.

The authors of the Kaiser study warned that the difficulty of separating the effects of marijuana and alcohol made for complications in their analysis. The subjects who smoked marijuana were much more inclined to be heavy drinkers than the non-users. This was because the heaviest-drinking subgroup of non-users of marijuana, namely tobacco smokers, was excluded. Also, no attempt was made to control for the use of other drugs, such as cocaine.

In conclusion, the leading health risks of marijuana appear to be (1) respiratory disease from smoking and (2) accidents resulting from mental impairment. Luckily, both can be greatly reduced by taking some precautions.

THE ACT OF SMOKING

Like tobacco, marijuana smoke is bad for the throat and lungs. Aside from their psychoactive ingredients, marijuana and tobacco smoke are chemically similar; both contain toxins that are known to be hazardous to the respiratory system. These chemicals have nothing to do with THC or other cannabinoids; they are non-psychoactive byproducts of leaf combustion. Among them are the carcinogenic compounds known as polycyclic aromatic hydrocarbons (PAHs), which are thought to be a major factor in smoking-related cancers. Marijuana tars are somewhat higher in PAHs than tobacco on a weight-for-weight basis, and have been shown to be carcinogenic in animal and human cell culture studies.

In addition to the solid tars, marijuana smoke includes gaseous toxins that are thought to be risk factors in heart and respiratory disease. Among these are hydrogen cyanide, carbon monoxide, nitrogen oxides, phenols, and volatile aldehydes.

Human studies have shown that heavy marijuana users have a higher risk of respiratory disease, including bronchitis, sore throat, and other infections. Oddly, the Kaiser study found that these risks were highest in users who had been using marijuana for less than 10 years, whereas longer-term users showed no greater risks than non-smokers. The authors suggested a possible explanation: users with respiratory problems may be more likely to quit early.

Although the Kaiser study was not large enough to detect smoking-related cancer, there is some circumstantial evidence to suggest that heavy pot smoking can cause cancer. Cancer specialists have reported a connection between marijuana smoking and cancers of the throat and oral cavity in younger males. Among patients who contract throat cancer before age 40, marijuana use appears to be even more prevalent than cigarette smoking, according to reports by Dr. Paul Donald, at the University of California at Davis, and by others.

Most, but not all, throat cancer victims also have other risk factors, particularly cigarette smoking and alcohol drinking. Pot smokers should definitely avoid alcohol and cigarettes, both of which aggravate the risks of throat cancer.

Cancer risks are directly dependent on total lifetime exposure. They're mostly of concern to long-term, heavy users who have smoked more than a joint per day for 15 or 20 years. They're not significant for patients who use marijuana occasionally, for a course of chemotherapy or for an occasional seizure.

MARIJUANA VERSUS TOBACCO

Marijuana is inherently safer than tobacco in that it does not contain nicotine, a powerful, addictive vasoconstrictor and stimulant that is known to promote circulatory disease.

A popular myth spread by "pothibitionists" is that one or two joints per day is equivalent to a pack-a-day cigarette habit. In fact, according to Dr. Donald Tashkin of UCLA, daily marijuana smokers show less evidence of respiratory damage than pack-a-day cigarette smokers. Undoubtedly, the reason for this is that marijuana smokers consume less material. A typical dose of marijuana is one or two joints per day, whereas cigarette smokers are likely to consume one or two packs of 20.

On the other hand, we have to adjust for the fact that marijuana smokers tend to inhale more deeply, exposing themselves to a greater quantity of smoke per puff. A study by Drs. Tashkin and T.-C. Wu found that marijuana smokers absorb between three and five times as much smoke toxins as tobacco smokers per weight smoked. Therefore, one gram of marijuana is equal to three to five grams of tobacco. Given that an average joint weighs 0.4 grams, about half as much as a cigarette, this means an average joint is equal to between 1.5 and 2.5 cigarettes.

Another difference between marijuana and tobacco is that tobacco smoke tends to penetrate more deeply into the lungs. For whatever reason, marijuana smoke tends to concentrate in the larger, upper air passageways of the lungs and throat, while tobacco penetrates to the smaller, lower passageways. One result of this is, apparently, that marijuana doesn't cause emphysema, a progressive, degenerative disease of the lower lungs that is linked to tobacco smoking. On the other hand, marijuana may be more apt to irritate the throat than cigarettes.

Marijuana smokers should probably abandon the practice of deeply inhaling and holding their breath. Studies have shown that this does little to increase THC absorption, but may substantially increase the respiratory hazards of smoking.

ACCIDENTS

The single greatest health concern for most marijuana users is the risk of accidents caused by impairment. Marijuana has adverse effects on psychomotor skills that are related to driving and other activities. Although the dangers of marijuana are less than those of drunken driving, they're still real. Contrary to the myth that no one has ever been hurt by using marijuana, there's no doubt that some accident fatalities have occurred. Such accidents result from careless, irresponsible use, which can be avoided with a proper understanding of marijuana's effects.

Studies have shown that marijuana adversely affects various driving skills, in particular tracking ability, or the ability to maintain a constant speed and distance from other cars; attentiveness; judgment of speed and distance; peripheral vision;

and coordination at complex tasks. Balance and muscle steadiness are also adversely affected.

Marijuana doesn't noticeably interfere with simple coordination or reaction time—for instance, the ability to put on the brakes quickly. However, it does hurt your coordination and reaction time at complex tasks, when decision making is needed—for instance, choosing whether to swerve right or left to avoid an obstacle, or whether to speed up or stop at a crossing when a speeding train is approaching. In general, marijuana is not as dangerous in routine driving as in emergency situations.

Off the road, the greatest danger of marijuana may be its adverse effect on short-term memory. Users may forget important safety procedures, leave the water or the stove turned on, lose their keys, and so on. Marijuana is to be avoided in jobs that require concentration, such as airline traffic control or operating complex machinery.

One of the most disconcerting effects of marijuana is that it makes familiar things seem strange. Drivers may suddenly find themselves lost in familiar neighborhoods, or forget to take the right freeway exit.

Fortunately, marijuana users are usually quite aware of their condition and tend to compensate for it. Most drivers tend to slow down under the influence of marijuana. In fact, many police consider slow driving to be a telltale sign of marijuana use. In this way, marijuana differs tremendously from alcohol, which tends to provoke speeding and reckless behavior.

In a recent study of marijuana and driving, National Highway Transportation Safety Administration (NHTSA) researchers concluded that marijuana produces a modest, dose-related reduction in road tracking performance, whose effects are "in no way unusual compared to many medicinal drugs." It found that even at higher doses, marijuana had smaller adverse effects on driving than alcohol at .08% blood alcohol content.

The legal threshold for driving under the influence of alcohol typically ranges from .08% to .10%.

Other accident studies have confirmed that marijuana is a smaller driving danger than alcohol. In another NHTSA study of 1,882 fatal driving accidents, alcohol was found in the blood of 51.5% of all victims, versus 6.7% for marijuana. Two thirds of the marijuana-using drivers also had alcohol in their systems. After analyzing the accidents in which marijuana alone was involved, NHTSA concluded that "there was no indication that marijuana by itself was a cause of fatal accidents."

On the other hand, the combination of alcohol and marijuana was definitely dangerous. Driving studies have found that the adverse effects of marijuana and other drugs are additive. In a California survey of young males killed in driving accidents, 80% of marijuana-related fatalities also involved alcohol. Obviously, marijuana users should avoid alcohol and other drugs.

Marijuana causes significant psychomotor impairment for the first couple of hours after smoking. After that, the effects fade. A few studies have detected subtle effects for four to eight hours, but these don't seem to be a major safety concern. One research team claimed to have found very subtle effects of marijuana for up to 24 hours on airline flight simulator tests, but other studies have not confirmed these effects.

If you've used marijuana recently, you may want to check yourself before driving. If you find yourself losing track of conversations, or forgetting what you were about to say, you're too stoned to drive. One simple test for motor coordination is to try to talk while standing on one foot. If you lose your balance, you're probably stoned. Another test is to extend your arms to both sides and close your eyes, then draw in each hand and try to touch your nose with your fingertip. If you miss, you're probably stoned.

INTOXICATION AND MENTAL IMPAIRMENT

For most users, the most important adverse effect of marijuana is mental impairment due to intoxication.

Marijuana seriously interferes with such mental skills as memorization, recall, attentiveness, tracking ability, and coordination at complex tasks. Many users have trouble trying to work, study, or perform difficult tasks while under its influence. Some users develop a tolerance to these effects after a period of chronic use, or learn to compensate and adjust their performance satisfactorily. Some folks manage to go about their everyday lives, more or less satisfactorily, under the continual influence of cannabis. Of course, some of them may be impaired in certain ways without knowing it.

Some people claim that marijuana actually improves their performance, especially at tasks requiring creativity, personal interaction, or rote, repetitive work where boredom is a problem. Scientific studies have failed to support these claims. Still, it's interesting that there was a time when mine and plantation owners in South America and Africa encouraged workers to take a cannabis break to boost morale and productivity!

Marijuana use has no detectable effect on normal intellectual performance when you're not under the influence. Some people have claimed that heavy use is linked to a decline in so-called "executive functioning," the ability to concentrate and focus your efforts on particular goals. Psychological tests generally do show that heavy pot users are more easily distracted and less attentive to maintaining a course of action.

In any case, problems of this kind are a matter of recreational abuse and aren't really relevant to medical users. Many patients find marijuana essential to their daily functioning, relieving them from the distractions of pain, discomfort, and debilitating suffering.

5

METHODS OF USING MARIJUANA AS MEDICINE

DOONESBURY
by Garry Trudeau

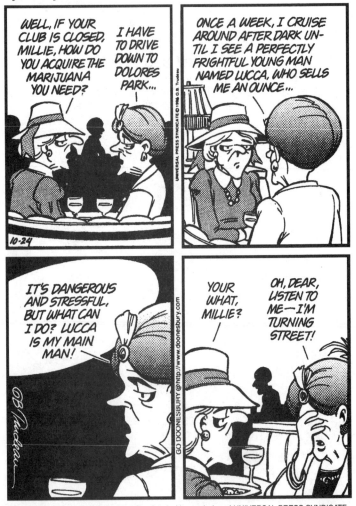

5

POTENCY OF PLANTS AND PLANT PARTS

Earlier, we mentioned briefly that different varieties and even different plants of the same variety may vary in potency. Different strains of marijuana have a wide range of effects. The pure genetic strains developed by indigenous peoples and traditional cultures are among the most effective for healing purposes. Certain Indica-type strains from the Afghani region and exotic Sativas from India and Thailand are outstanding for medicinal use, but they are not readily available in the U.S. The most promising strains of marijuana which are available are the Indica/Sativa hybrids. These strains are the result of years of home based breeding experiments by people from all over the world.

INDICAS

Indicas have a broad set of characteristics but are generally body-oriented and muscle relaxing. They are helpful for people with sleep disorders. Some strains allow a person to become a bit detached and relaxed, so emotional and physical stresses can come to rest and be accepted. Even something as basic as using an Indica with a hot bath or sauna will alleviate a great deal of stress associated with illness, enabling many people to get rest and deep sleep where otherwise it would not be possible without the use of more toxic, expensive, synthetic pharmaceuticals.

High quality Indica strains may also help when patients work with massage, techniques such as Rolfing, Hatha Yoga, and Shiatsu. Chiropractic work seems to be accepted deeper into the body with longer lasting benefits for the patient.

If the chosen therapy and a small amount of marijuana is combined with a hot bath before and after, the results can be an overall feeling of relaxed well-being which can be of tremendous support to one who is ill. This benefit may not be duplicated by synthetic pharmaceuticals.

Some Indica strains are so "heavy" in feeling that they induce lethargy and make effective functioning and clear thinking difficult. Such strains may be more appropriate for bedridden patients. "Heaviness" is aggravated by excessive dosages and patients should begin with small amounts so as not to overdo it.

SATIVAS

Sativas are more "heady," inspirational and "focused." Some Sativas are well suited for more refined healing practices where full attention and participation are required: therapies which incorporate breathing exercises, internal imagery, visualization or creative arts, music writing, and dance. Doing something creative that you like doing can be an effective stimulus for staying alive and getting well. Creative engagement will also greatly serve a dying person who still has the urge to express his or her heart and share creative ways with loved ones.

Good Sativa strains are more difficult to get access to. Due to lower weight yields, longer growing seasons and finicky growing requirements they are not generally the choice of growers.

If someone feels very disconnected from their body, or is extremely underweight, Indicas might be better recommended as Sativas tend to be heady, mental and abstract. If a person is already inclined to forget they have a body or if they are having trouble staying connected to body functions, Sativas won't offer as much help as good Indica.

For other people, Sativas can stimulate bodily life-force feelings by energizing one's relationship to physical activity. This can make the physically active part of life a happy and pleasurable experience again. Some Indica/Sativa varieties also seem well suited for highly demanding physical activities. For someone who is ill to feel again the joy of his or her body moving in a ball sport, swimming or exercising, or even just working around the home, is a blessing that energizes and stimulates body functions and literally brings more life in the body.

The new hybrids show some of cannabis' full potential. Indica strains' heaviness has been lessened while the best qualities and characteristics have been left intact. This has been combined with the more subtle, high-energy Sativa characteristics. The results can be highly effective for medicinal purposes. It seems likely that specific varieties can be developed to uniquely address specific illnesses.

Environmental factors also play a part in the potency of the bud. Growing conditions, weather, and care affect the quality of marijuana, just as with flowers and vegetables.

Different parts of the marijuana plant have different potencies. THC is found in glands that grow on the surface of the plant's stem and leaves. They are most concentrated on the tiny leaves and stems surrounding and inside the clusters of female flowers. Larger leaves from this area are usually picked off (manicured) once the buds have been taken off the plant. These leaves are called trim, and contain less THC than the smaller leaves and organs surrounding the flower. The large fan, or sun, leaves contain even fewer glands and are considerably less potent than the flowers or the trim. They are usually used for ingestion rather than smoking, because they are so harsh and only mildly potent.

In recent years, drug warriors have tried to scare the public about the supposed hazards of more potent marijuana. Ignoring the advantages of higher-potency marijuana for reducing smoke inhalation, drug czar Lee Brown falsely claimed that potency in 1995 was 40 times greater than in the Sixties, making marijuana a whole new drug. In fact, average potency has increased only modestly, by a factor of 2 or 3, while the range of potencies available has remained the same. High-potency preparations, including hashish, hash oil, special strains, and extracts have been widely available since the nineteenth century.

High-potency formulations have been especially popular for medical use. Up through the 1930s, when cannabis was available over the counter in pharmacies throughout the U.S., it was sold in alcohol-based tinctures of 25% potency. Recommended doses were measured in drops.

On balance, high-potency sinsemilla and concentrated preparations are preferable for most medical users, to protect them from harmful smoke. When inhalation is not necessary, oral ingestion is better.

CONCENTRATING GRASS

Sinsemilla (seedless) marijuana buds retail for hundreds of dollars per ounce—up to several thousand dollars per pound—and usually contain between 4% and 8% THC. The large fan leaves contain between 1% and 2% THC; they retail for only $100 to $300 per pound. The trim leaves contain 2% to 3% THC and retail for $200 to $500 per pound. You can see that the leaves are much more economical than the buds and are truly the best buy. The only problem is that they are harsh on the throat and not pleasant to smoke.

The solution to this dilemma is to concentrate the THC so that only the potent part—the glands—is used. There are several ways to do this.

SCREENING

The easiest screen to use is a silkscreen or, even better, a steel or plastic mesh screen with 100 or 125 lines to the inch. The spaces in the screen are large enough to allow the glands to drop through. The vegetable material stays on the top. The yield depends on the quality of the material you started with.

To use a screen, stretch it tight and then rub bone-dry vegetative material against it. To get the vegetation dry, just place it in a microwave oven. It need not be broken up. The longer the material is rubbed, the more glands will fall through. The process is analogous to olive pressing, in which

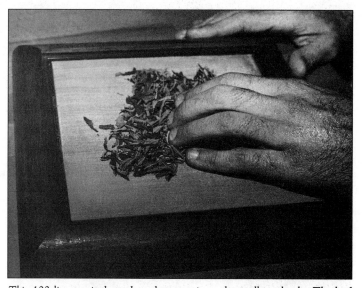

This 100-line-per-inch steel mesh screen is used to collect glands. The leaf shown here is rubbed against the screen. The glands are knocked off and fall below so they can be collected. The screen can also be used as a rolling tray.

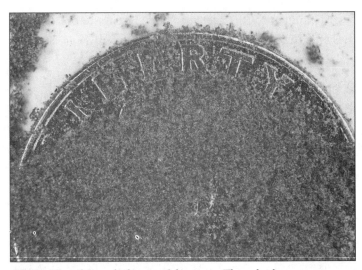

Glands collected from the bottom of the screen. These glands are very concentrated, so they're very potent.

the longer the press, the lower the quality of the oil, because more impurities are pressed out. As marijuana is rubbed, a higher percentage of extraneous vegetative matter falls through as the process continues.

If the marijuana is rubbed for a long time, then, more THC-containing glands fall through the screen and more vegetative matter falls through as well. Though this makes the material less desirable for smoking, the additional vegetative matter is not significant when it's ingested. For eating, a larger yield, even if in a less concentrated form, is the goal.

Rubbing glands for smoking requires a little finesse. The very first screening produces the best 'kief'—unpressed hashish. Glands that fall through the screen can be smoked in a pipe, added to a joint, or ingested. They are extremely potent, so only a little bit is needed.

WATER SCREENING

THC glands are heavier than water and sink, whereas most vegetative material is lighter and floats. This makes it easy to concentrate the glands as long as they can be detached from the vegetative material. The resulting "kief" is very clean and concentrated. Before water screening, the grass can be screened mechanically, though it doesn't have to be. Since the glands are literally washed, pollutants, molds, and fungi are rinsed away.

Whole marijuana is put in a jar and cold water is added. Then the mix is shaken for a few minute or so. The vegetative material stays on top and is removed. The THC-containing glands fall to the bottom. They are rinsed out of the jar and dried.

Don't use warm or even tepid water. With cold water, the glands remain rigid and brittle. When warm water is used, they become soft and sticky; this makes them much harder to work with.

The glands are very powerful. Only a pinch is needed in a pipe bowl to provide relief. They can also be swallowed in capsules or eaten in food.

One medical user uses the THC-bearing glands in cooking. She has a small container of the substance and uses a tiny spoon to add it to her food.

METHODS OF TAKING THE DOSE

Cannabis is either smoked or eaten. Each method of use has its advantages and disadvantages. The two methods can be used separately or together.

Smoking is the most common way people use marijuana. It is very fast-acting. Within a few seconds of inhaling, THC reaches the alveoli in the lungs and is absorbed into the blood system. As soon as it reaches the receptors in the brain and organs, usually in less than a minute, its effects can be felt.

After the effect begins, the high continues to grow quickly for about 15 minutes and deepens a little for another 10 to 20 minutes. After this peak, the high begins to fade and is gone within one to three hours. This helps relieve symptoms quickly. It also makes it easier to determine how much to use. Smoked marijuana is especially advantageous when there is a problem with nausea or lack of appetite, since you don't have to eat it.

Lower-quality marijuana is felt as quickly as high-quality, but it reaches its peak more quickly and lasts a shorter time. Both the individual's susceptibility to marijuana and the marijuana quality affect the high.

Ingestion produces somewhat different effects from inhalation because material that is eaten is first processed by the liver before it reaches the brain. In the liver, the material is converted to 11-hydroxy-THC, a metabolite that is some four to five times more psychoactively potent than ordinary THC. Because 11-hydroxy-THC is not produced when marijuana is smoked, eating and smoking produce different pharmacological effects.

Ingested marijuana takes longer to be felt and its effects last longer. The long-lasting nature of ingested marijuana can be very helpful. Some people regulate their conditions by eating small amounts of marijuana. They barely feel any effect from the drug except for the relief of their symptoms.

The major drawback of ingestion is that the effective dose can be hard to predict. Depending on the state of your digestive system, the contents of your stomach, and other unpredictable factors, a given oral dose may be absorbed more or less easily. It may take several hours to take full effect. As we've pointed out, this makes it difficult to gauge exactly how great a dose you have taken, so it's hard to know beforehand how much to eat.

One of the advantages of ingestion is that people usually use relatively low-grade marijuana, such as leaf, which is considered a by-product of bud production.

OINTMENTS AND POULTICES

Some patients apply marijuana externally, or topically, to the skin in the form of ointments, lotions, or poultices, for treatment of swollen joints and other ailments.

It's not clear how well, if at all, topical treatment works. Indeed, according to Dr. Mahmoud El Sohly, a leading authority on cannabinoid chemistry, there is no known method for transporting THC or other cannabinoids through the skin. Instead, Dr. El Sohly has proposed using rectal suppositories, which he claims are a better way of delivering cannabinoids to the system.

Nevertheless, some patients claim they find benefits in direct application. Tom says he has gotten relief from rheumatism by rubbing his joints with an ointment made from 4 ounces of marijuana leaf soaked in 16 ounces of oil. He applies the ointment with alcohol.

At the turn of the century, cannabis was used as a topical ingredient in remedies for corns (either as an anesthetic or as an antiviral agent). Topical cannabis applications have also been used in folk medicine in India and Latin America. One popular treatment for arthritis in the Mexican-American community is to wrap the joints in a poultice, or bandage, of cannabis leaves. In order to promote extraction of the cannabinoids, the leaves are soaked in alcohol. Aside from the problem of obtaining enough leaves to make a poultice, it's not clear that this practice is anything more than a placebo.

INHALING/SMOKING MARIJUANA

KILLING PATHOGENS

Many doctors recommend that patients with impaired immune systems be sure to sterilize all marijuana that they use, whether it's smoked or eaten. They may be saying this as a matter of course rather than because there is a real danger of infection. However, a few people have become sick from infected marijuana. You would expect the pathogens to be killed by burning, because the smoke from marijuana is a pyrolytic product, the result of burning, so any pathogens that may be in it should die in the burn. However, the smoke does pass through cooler, unburned material, so pathogens can enter the smoke stream.

Though the chance of infection is low, it's best for people with injured immune systems to make sure all pathogens are killed before they use marijuana. There are several ways to do this. These include cooking and using a microwave. Some people prefer using a microwave because its beams first dry the grass, then kill any pathogens in the material.

If an oven or a toaster oven is used, the grass can quickly get burned and the THC can quickly evaporate or be destroyed. The oven should be kept at a temperature of 160 degrees, which will kill most microorganisms but will not destroy the THC. The grass needs to be baked for only a few minutes.

If marijuana is cooked in a liquid such as a broth or sauce that simmers or boils, it is sterilized by the heat. Marijuana used in recipes that are not heated to boiling is also safe. When the heat during cooking reaches 160 degrees, it causes pasteurization, in which most pathogens are killed. Pasteurized milk has been through the same process.

PREPARING MARIJUANA FOR SMOKING

To burn evenly and smoke well, marijuana should be free of sticks and seeds. Most domestically grown marijuana is sinsemilla—from the Spanish sin (without) and semilla (seeds)—and, of course, is seedless. Imported marijuana, including many grades of Mexican, often contains a considerable number of seeds. These must be removed before the marijuana is smoked, or they will pop when they get hot. This can send a hard-burning particle, or at least a very hot one, in any direction, but usually toward the most recent clothing purchase that is in the immediate area. Burning seed also releases an acrid smoke that most people find foul. Some even find that burning seed gives them a mild headache.

The best way to remove seeds from marijuana is to break several marijuana buds up by cutting them with a pair of scissors, so that all the seeds are released from the vegetation. Remove any small twigs at this stage. Don't try to remove the seeds at this point, though; it will be too tedious.

To remove seeds, most people use their fingers, but when they do this many of the glands are removed from the pot and stick to the skin, removing some of the active ingredient. After the first layer of glands has stuck to the skin, glands that they come in contact with also stick. This is all right if you're manicuring large amounts. After a while, a layer builds up that is thick enough to be rubbed off the fingers. This mixture of glands and human oils is a form of hashish and can be smoked. Since it is a concentration of the glands, it is much more potent than the buds.

If you're cleaning only enough for a few joints, however, only a thin layer of glands builds up. It does not easily peel or rub off the skin, although it's easily removed using a tissue or soap and water. Either way, it's lost.

There is a partial solution. Use scissors to cut the buds up. Not as many glands will stick to the scissors as to your fingers. The glands accumulate on the scissors and can eventually be scraped off. Still, many of the glands never make it to the joint.

Removing the seeds from marijuana is best done using a "rolling tray," which can be as simple as a shoe-box top, a plate, or a screen device. You place the grass at one end of the tray. The tray is held at a slight angle, with the grass at the lower end, and using a business card, a playing card (not the Queen of Spades), or a canceled credit card, you push the vegetation and seeds toward the top, up the slope. The heavy, slightly oval seeds will roll down while the vegetation stays in place.

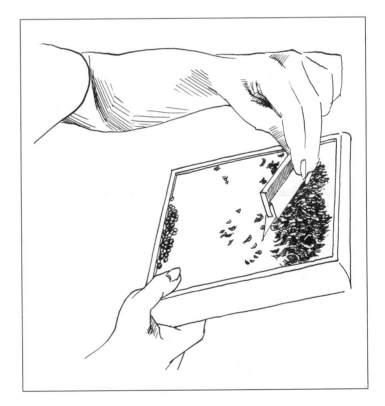

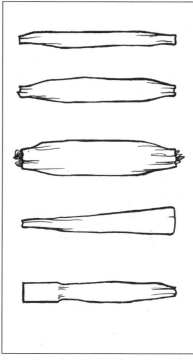

Joints, top to bottom: Regular joint, Dealer's joint, Grower's joint, European joint, and joint with filter.

Continue doing this until the seeds stop rolling out. Then look for any seeds that may be hidden and gently nudge them to start them rolling. When all the seeds have been removed, the marijuana is ready to use.

Sinsemilla is handled differently. Since there are no seeds, the buds don't need to be broken up for cleaning, but just into small enough pieces to roll into a joint or place in the bowl of a pipe. If you use a photographer's loupe, you can see the glands on the surfaces of the leaves. The heads of these glands contain the THC. Be aware that these glands break away from the leaf at the slightest provocation, such as a touch or even a strong wind. This lowers the amount left to use.

METHODS OF SMOKING

JOINTS

Joints (marijuana cigarettes) are probably the most common way people smoke marijuana. They are convenient to use, are easy to carry and dispose of, leave no paraphernalia trail, and are easily shared. Many people get oral satisfaction from

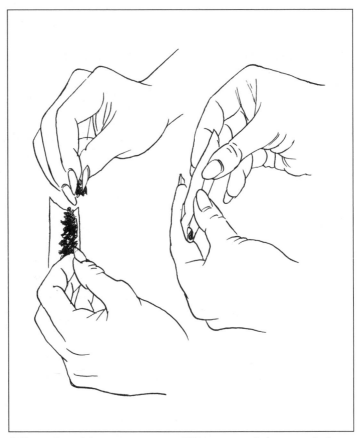

Rolling a Joint. Marijuana is put into fold in paper with the gummed edge on the far side. Side closest to body is folded under the other side of the paper.

toking on a joint in the same way as they might if smoking a cigarette.

Before marijuana can be rolled into a joint, it must be broken into small pieces so that it will be evenly distributed. This is best done using scissors.

Joints can be rolled either using a hand rolling machine or completely by hand. In different countries, they're rolled in different ways. The two that are most familiar to us are the

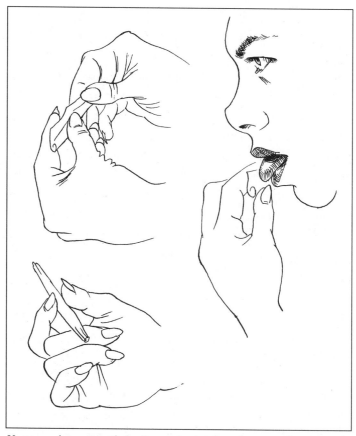

Keeping a firm grip with forefinger, the thumb pushes upward, causing the paper to roll. Tap down on glued section, lick gummed end and fasten.

American joint and the Dutch spliff. (See illustrations above for instructions on how to roll a joint and a spliff.) People who have difficulty hand-rolling joints can use one of the machine rollers available in some smoke shops. Joints comes in many sizes.

After the joint is rolled, it is placed in the mouth, similarly to a cigarette; breath is drawn in through the joint so that the airstream picks up the smoke.

PIPES

Pipes have grown in popularity and many people prefer them to joints. There are several reasons. Unlike joints, they use no paper or glue, so the smoke contains no impurities. They usually have small bowls, so that just a small amount of bud can be used. This prevents waste from sidestream smoke.

There are innumerable pipe designs, ranging from the most basic implements to true works of art. No matter how stylish the pipe is, it should have an easy draw, be comfortable to use, and be easy to clean.

Pipes have been made from every conceivable material. In a pipe shop, you're likely to see glass, wood, metal, and plastic pipes. There have been no studies specifically checking residues from heated pipes, but it is generally agreed that glass, stainless steel, and brass are inert. Burning wood may produce some fumes, but hardwoods require a greater heat than that in the bowl to start smoldering. All plastic pipes are suspect and should be avoided.

Some pipes feature a "carburetor," which is a small hole in the air chamber located past the bowl. The carburetor is held shut while the bowl is being lit and the smoke drawn. Then, when the carburetor is released the free air drawn in allows the smoke to be drawn into the lungs more quickly.

WATERPIPES AND BONGS

Waterpipes work by drawing the smoke through a water filter. This both cools the smoke and removes particles from it, making the draw smoother. Just as with conventional pipes, people have applied a tremendous amount of ingenuity to the design of waterpipes. There are an incredible number of styles and designs.

Most pipes have a bowl on top of a stem that ends below the waterline. The air tube is above the water. When you draw on the tube, air is pulled through the bowl, the stem, and the water, so the air is filtered by the water. The smaller the size of the bubbles and the greater the length of the tube of water through which they pass, the more filtering the water does.

A bong is a specialized type of waterpipe; it has a large chamber in which the smoke is held before it is inhaled. When the carburetor is released, a large amount of smoke is inhaled quickly.

Although many folks prefer to use waterpipes because of the cooler, smoother smoke they produce, it's not clear that waterpipes are actually healthier for the lungs. The reason is that waterpipes can absorb even more THC than they do other, carcinogenic compounds. As a result, users may end up consuming more harmful smoke toxins in order to absorb the same dose of THC.

A smoking device study, sponsored by California NORML and MAPS (the Multidisciplinary Association for Psychedelic Studies), found that waterpipes absorb at least 30% more cannabinoids than carcinogenic tars. Therefore, in order to obtain the same effective dose of THC, a smoker would end up taking in 30% more tars from a waterpipe than from an unfiltered joint. The more thorough the water mixing, the lower the proportion of THC to total tars. This suggests that water filtration may actually be counterproductive!

However, the study did not examine the vapor phase of the smoke, which contains a number of toxic gases, such as carbon monoxide, aldehydes, phenols, and hydrogen cyanide. Some of these are quite water soluble, and are likely to be screened out by waterpipes. If so, waterpipes may still have some health benefits.

Another smoke filtration strategy is to inhale the smoke through a cigarette filter. Though there are a number of ingenious devices to accomplish this, they offer no advantages.

The NORML / MAPS study found that cigarette filters had the same drawbacks as waterpipes, increasing the ratio of tars to THC by some 30%. Unlike waterpipes, there is no reason to expect that cigarette filters would reduce toxic gases. Worst of all, though, the study found that they eliminated fully 60% of the THC from the smoke stream. This means you would have to smoke 2.5 times as much marijuana through a cigarette filter to get the same dose of THC as with an unfiltered joint!

That's why cigarette filters are counterproductive.

VAPORIZERS

The most promising way of eliminating marijuana smoke toxins is through vaporization. In theory, cannabinoids can be vaporized from marijuana without producing any pyrolytic compounds by holding the temperature below the point of combustion, at which hydrocarbons in the leaf would begin to oxidize. Cannabinoids vaporize around 185 to 190 degrees Centigrade, while carcinogenic aromatic hydrocarbons begin to form around 560 degrees Centigrade. If you hold the temperature around 185 to 190 degrees Centigrade, then, it should be possible to produce pure cannabinoid vapors without any harmful smoke toxins.

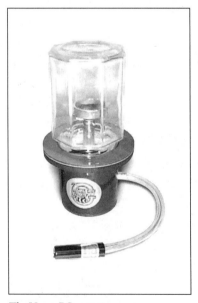

The Hemp BC vaporizer.

Unfortunately, the development of vaporizers has been impeded by the U.S. paraphernalia laws, which outlaw the sale of devices for smoking marijuana. (Waterpipes and other pipes are exempt because they can conceivably be used for tobacco.)

In the early 1980s, a vaporizer known as the Tilt was briefly marketed and advertised in High Times. The Tilt was tested at MIT, where it was found to produce 80% less tars and 80% more THC than a standard pipe. It also produced no carbon monoxide. This pipe would be ideal for using lower-quality marijuana, such as leaf, as well as for extracting THC from the best buds.

Unfortunately, the paraphernalia laws put the company out of business just as it was getting started. Still. a pipe such as this can be constructed at home. Plans for a homemade vaporizer by "Dr. Lunglife" are available from California NORML.

Recently, other vaporizers have been developed for sale abroad. In Canada a model, with an electric heating element, is sold by Hemp BC in Vancouver, British Columbia.

The NORML / MAPS smoking study tested two vaporizers: a homemade device made from a paint stripper and an electric model imported from Canada. Both produced modestly less tar per unit THC than the unfiltered joint, though neither came close to matching the Tilt. More disturbingly, they yielded less than 30% as much total THC as the unfiltered joint. Clearly, more developmental work needs to be done on vaporizers.

USE HIGH-POTENCY MARIJUANA

Until the development of better smoking devices, the easiest way to reduce noxious smoke toxins is simply to use stronger pot. High-grade sinsemilla with a potency of 8% will deliver four times as much THC per puff as low-grade "ditchweed" with a potency of 2%. By carefully adjusting your intake to the dose of THC, you can greatly reduce your exposure to harmful tars by using more potent material.

The limitations of this method are:

1) Higher-potency cannabis typically has lower levels of CBD, so it may not be as good if CBD is what you need. Such problems can be avoided by using high-potency extracts prepared from low-potency, higher-CBD marijuana.

2) More attention may be needed to avoid overdosing with extremely high-potency varieties.

6

COOKING WITH MARIJUANA

DOONESBURY
by Garry Trudeau

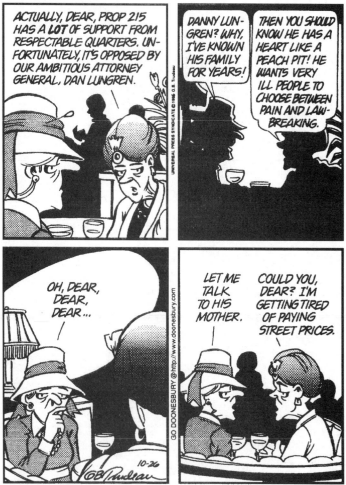

6

REDUCING THE "WEEDY" FLAVOR OF MARIJUANA

There are some recipes that just don't go well with the strong flavor of marijuana, which comes from its water-soluble compounds. However, these can be extracted, leaving the leaf with a much less intense flavor.

Use whole leaf. Place the marijuana in a bowl, being sure not to pack it too tightly. Add tepid water and let the marijuana soak for about half an hour. The water will change color as much of the chlorophyll and other pigments is dissolved. Pour off the water. The marijuana is now ready to be used as is, or it can be dried and powdered.

After pouring off the water and removing the marijuana, you'll probably see a tan-colored residue at the bottom of the bowl. This substance consists of glands that have fallen off the leaf. It can be dried and is very potent. This process is similar to the "water screening" process we described earlier.

DRY PREPARATION

This process can be used with any form of marijuana—buds, trim, or leaf. The marijuana may have gone through the water process described above or not, but it must be very dry.

Marijuana is ground using a blender. First the marijuana is dried until it is crisp and breaks easily in your fingers. This can be done in a microwave oven or a food dehydrator. Sensitive ovens with a setting of 100 degrees Fahrenheit also work well. Once the marijuana is dry, place it in a blender on high speed.

If only a small amount is being processed, a coffee grinder may be more convenient. Grind the marijuana until it is powdery. Don't open the top right away, because the dust, which contains the THC-bearing glands, has to settle first. This takes about five minutes. Once it has been ground, the marijuana is sifted through a strainer. This is done to remove unchopped leaf veins. It should be done in a room with little air circulation, using a high-walled bowl, not a plate, so that the ultra-light THC glands don't drift into the atmosphere. Once the marijuana is ground and sifted, it is ready to use in cooking.

ALCOHOL OR OIL EXTRACT PREPARATION

The most popular way of cooking with grass is to dissolve the THC in alcohol, butter, or oil. This can be done after soaking the marijuana in water. The color of the alcohol, butter, or oil doesn't become as deep and the flavor doesn't get as intense.

Making an alcohol mix is very easy. Just add the grass to any 80-proof or stronger alcohol. The theory is that the stronger the alcohol, the more THC will be dissolved in it. Though this theory has not been tested, we suspect that 80-proof (40%) alcohol is strong enough to dissolve all the THC. Most of the THC dissolves within a few hours. Within two days, the process is complete. Mixing or shaking the alcohol helps this process along.

Be careful to measure the amount of marijuana you add so that the dose per unit of alcohol can be calculated. For instance, a fifth of alcohol is equal to 26 ounces. An ounce of marijuana is equal to 28 grams. Slightly less than one ounce of marijuana soaked in one fifth of alcohol would make 26 one-gram-per-ounce servings. If the amount of marijuana were doubled, a one-gram dose would be contained in one-half ounce of liquor.

Whole leaves can be added to the alcohol and are just as effective as ground marijuana, though their bulkiness makes them hard to stuff into a narrow-necked bottle. The alcohol can always be poured into a wide-necked jar for processing. This way, more leaf can be processed too. Once the processing is complete, the leaf is easily removed from the alcohol. Be sure to press the alcohol from the leaf before you discard it. (If the leaf is placed in a narrow-necked bottle, it doesn't have to be removed and can be discarded with the empty bottle.)

Some people prefer to add ground marijuana to the alcohol. It's less messy, easier to handle, and much less bulky, so a greater concentration is possible. To remove the remains, just pour the mixture out through a coffee filter.

MARIJUANA COOKING OIL

THC-containing oil is also easy to make. Just add the marijuana to any vegetable oil the same way as described for alcohol. Within a few days, the THC dissolves in the oil.

1 pint olive oil
64 grams dry weight (approx. 2¼ oz.) washed ground leaf

Place oil and leaf in a container. Let it sit for three days or more in a cool dark place. Strain through a fine tea strainer to remove the grounds. Then press the leaf oil between two strainers to squeeze the oil out. Each half tablespoon of oil will contain a one-gram portion.

An alternative method of using the oil is to keep the leaf in the liquid. Before using, shake or stir the oil to mix the marijuana throughout, then measure out the amount desired.

MARIJUANA BUTTER (OR MARGARINE)

Marijuana butter takes a little more effort, but is still quite easy to make.

2 sticks butter (8 oz.)
16 ounces water
32 grams leaf

Heat the water and butter together in a pot. Add the marijuana and stir occasionally. Keep simmering for about a half hour. Then remove the leaf from the mixture. Put the pot in the refrigerator. The butter will solidify at the top of the water. Discard the water. The marijuana butter is now ready to use in your favorite recipe, or just as a spread on some bread. One half tablespoon of butter equals a one-gram portion.

Dave's Famous Cookies, formerly sold at the S.F. Cannabis Buyers' Club, are made using a simple technique. Dave prepares the marijuana by removing all stems, then powders it using a blender. Then he strains it to remove any leaf stems. He adds this to a mixture of butter and oil, heats it until it simmers, and then adds the oil with the marijuana to an almond cookie batter with chocolate chips.

We once tasted a truly delicious marijuana cake prepared by an acquaintance. He confided his secret: shortbread mix and marijuana rum. Certainly marijuana can be added to any cake or cookie mix, or you can use your own favorite recipe. You can use an alcohol or butter extract to add THC or, in some cases, add the marijuana directly to the mix.

Spicy corn bread was served at a recent dinner given by some S.F. Buyers' Club members. The recipe was taken right from the box, except that powdered marijuana was added. Each square contained about ⅛ gram of leaf. The hosts realized that guests would be eating more than one piece, so they kept the concentration low.

Many marijuana recipes use chocolate and coffee. These two flavors mask the marijuana taste well. Probably the best-known recipe is the famous "marijuana brownie" first popularized in Alice B. Toklas's 1930s cookbook.

The following recipes, which have been developed by medical users, are delicious—with or without the marijuana.

BEVERAGES

LHASSI (FOR ONE)

1 cup yogurt
1 cup crushed ice
Sugar, honey, or other sweetening to taste
Tiny pinch powdered cardamom (optional)
Tiny pinch powdered cloves (optional)
Few drops rosewater (optional)
1 portion marijuana butter or oil

Place all ingredients in a blender. Blend on the high setting until all the ice is thoroughly mixed in. Very refreshing on a hot day.

MARIJUANA LIQUEUR

1 pint liqueur (16 ounces)
8 grams (dry weight) whole presoaked leaf

Place the marijuana in a covered jar with the liqueur. Store in a cool, dark place until you remember it, but for at least three days. Pour and serve. You may wish to remove the leaves for aesthetic reasons.

Each ounce of liqueur is one half-gram serving.

MARIJUANA MILK

Heat a glass of milk or soy milk over a low flame on the stove or in a microwave oven. When it is warm, add one portion or more of water-treated marijuana. Keep the mixture warm, just below simmering, for half an hour. Strain the mix and discard the leaf. This milk can be used for cooking or drinking, or mixed with cereal.

DESSERTS

THE ULTIMATE GOURMET BROWNIE

6 oz. high-quality bittersweet chocolate
½ cup marijuana butter
4 tbsp chocolate syrup
2 tbsp unsweetened cocoa
1 tsp almond extract
4 egg whites, beaten fluffy
¾ cup sugar
⅛ tsp salt
½ cup flour
1 tsp baking powder

Melt chocolate, chocolate syrup, and cocoa over low heat, stirring constantly. Remove from the heat and stir in butter, oil, and egg whites. Mix thoroughly. Add salt, flour, sugar, and baking powder and blend completely. Pour into an 8" square baking pan and place in a preheated 350-degree oven for 30 minutes.

Of course, you can add nuts, coconut, or chocolate chips to the mix before you bake it. This makes sixteen 2" square brownies.

We discovered this great recipe for carrot cake in Tom Flower's book, *Marijuana Herbal Cookbook*. He kindly allowed us to reprint it here.

TOM'S CARROT CAKE

6 oz. butter
¼–½ oz. marijuana leaf
1 cup finely grated carrot
¾ cup brown sugar
¾ cup milk
2 large eggs
½ cup shredded coconut
1 tsp grated orange peel
1 tsp ginger
1¾ cup flour
1 tbsp baking powder

Beat softened butter and marijuana leaf. Add the carrot, sugar, milk, eggs, coconut, orange peel, and ginger. When this is thoroughly mixed, sift in flour and baking powder.

When everything is thoroughly mixed, pour the batter into an 8" square baking pan. Bake for 45 minutes at 325 degrees. This makes 16 slices.

CHOCOLATE PUDDING

You can prepare commercial chocolate pudding from a package (if you don't mind the list of ingredients in it)! This is how to do it:

1 package chocolate pudding mix
4 portions marijuana butter, oil, alcohol, or ground leaf

Prepare the pudding as directed. Add marijuana or extract to the mix when you add the milk or soy milk. For good portion control, pour into serving dishes while the pudding is still warm.

You can also make pudding for yourself. Here's another great recipe from Tom Flower's *Marijuana Herbal Cookbook*.

MILE HIGH CHOCOLATE PUDDING

Mix together:

¼ cup water
3 tbsp cornstarch

Set aside.
Whisk together in a saucepan:

1 egg (optional)
2 cups milk or soy milk
1 to 4 teaspoons of marijuana leaf or .5 to 2 grams of
   sinsemilla flowers
3 tbsp sugar
6 tbsp cocoa

Heat on low, stirring occasionally to keep it from sticking to the bottom of the pan. Just before the mix boils, stir the cornstarch and water and pour the blend into the mixture, stirring quickly until the mixture thickens. Serve hot or cold.

SAUCES

TOMATO SAUCE FROM A JAR

Marijuana can be simply prepared with a commercial tomato sauce. Take a half jar of sauce and add about 2 grams of nice-quality leaf in a pouch made of nylon netting, which can be bought at a home brew store. Push this into the tomato sauce (which should contain oil) and heat the mix in the microwave until boiling. Let the mix sit for about an hour, stirring about every 15 minutes. Then heat it up again, remove the pouch, and serve pasta for four.

TOMATO-VEGETABLE SAUCE

(Makes about 1 quart, or 8 servings)

2 lb. fresh plum tomatoes
1 large onion (5–6 oz.)
4 large cloves garlic (1 oz.)
1 large red pepper
1 small green pepper
2 stalks Swiss chard or ½ cup fresh spinach (optional)
3 tablespoons olive oil
2–6 level tsp finely chopped marijuana leaf
1 teaspoon Italian seasoning
1 tsp lecithin granules
½ tsp dried basil
¼ tsp salt
⅛ tsp black pepper

Dice onion, pepper, and Swiss chard stalks into ⅛-inch pieces, using knife or food processor. Grind garlic, using a press. Chop the tomatoes into one-inch cubes and cut the Swiss chard leaves into two-inch squares.

Heat saucepan on medium high, add oil, let it heat up, and then add chopped onions, garlic, and Swiss chard stalks. Fry until the onions are golden. Reduce the heat to low and let the pan cool. Add pressed garlic and marijuana, then stir into the vegetable oil mix for a minute or two. Add tomatoes and top with Swiss chard or spinach leaves. Cover and simmer for 15 minutes, stirring occasionally, until the tomatoes lose their firmness. Remove cover to let some of the water boil off and add lecithin. Stir occasionally. The sauce is ready in 10 to 20 minutes. This sauce can be served as is with the chunky vegetables. (For some recipes, you may prefer to grind the sauce in a blender.)

SOUP

NONDAIRY CREAMY CHICKEN VEGETABLE SOUP

(Makes twelve 8-oz. servings)

1½ *quarts water*
1 *skinless boneless chicken breast (1 lb.)*
1 *carrot*
1 *medium-size creamer or masher potato*
1 *small onion*
1 *small parsnip*
1 *small turnip*
1 *small red pepper*
1 *small leek*
4 *cloves garlic*
2 *tablespoons chopped parsley*
2 *bay leaves*
½ *tomato (optional)*
¼ *cup fresh or frozen corn kernels (optional)*
½ *tsp salt*

½ *tsp lecithin*
¼ *tsp Italian or chicken seasoning*
12 *portions marijuana leaf, alcohol, or oil*

Boil water. Chop all the vegetables into one-inch pieces. Add all ingredients to the water. Bring to a boil. Lower heat to simmer. Add marijuana. Turn heat off after one hour. Let cool to a comfortable temperature. Remove half the chicken and bay leaves. Chop all other ingredients in a blender. Cut up chicken pieces and add to soup.

VEGETABLES

MASHED POTATOES

(*Makes four 6½-oz servings*)

1¼ **lb. *hot, peeled, cooked creamed or boiled potatoes***
¼ *cup whole or 2% milk*
2 *ounces chervil cheese (or substitute creamy cottage, feta,*
    ricotta, or blue cheese)
4 *portions marijuana butter (1–2 ounces)*
2 *teaspoons chopped parsley*
1 *raw egg white*
¼ *teaspoon garlic granules or 2 cloves pressed garlic (*½ *oz.)*
½ *teaspoon fine herbs (or to taste)*
½ *teaspoon salt*
⅛ *teaspoon black pepper*
Dash *cayenne pepper or 1 squirt hot sauce (optional)*

While the potatoes are cooking, heat the milk, butter, cheese, garlic, and spices in a saucepan under low heat, stirring constantly until smooth. When the potatoes are soft, drain them and put them back into the cooking pot. Add the cheese mixture and egg white. Whip the potatoes, using an electric mixer or hand masher.

CHOW MEIN

(Serves 4)

½ cup water chestnuts
1 cup bok choy
6 green onions
½ cup bean sprouts
¼ cup broccoli flowers
¼ cup finely chopped green and red peppers
1 cup tofu
Seasonings to taste: Ginger, garlic, mustard, curry, turmeric,
   and lemon grass

SAUCE

1 tbsp soy sauce
2 tsp corn starch
1 tsp oil
¾ cup water
4 grams marijuana
Seasonings to taste

Peel water chestnuts or use canned ones. Chop into thin slices.
Cut bok choy into ¼-inch slices, set aside green parts. Cut
green onions, separating white from green, then chop the green
into ½-inch pieces and chop the white into ¼-inch pieces.
Cut broccoli into small pieces. Cut tofu into ½-inch pieces. In
a hot skillet or wok, place bok choy whites, green onion
whites, peppers, and broccoli. Fry for 2 minutes and set aside.
Put bean sprouts and all the greens in a pan along with a few
tablespoons of water and let steam in pan for 2–3 minutes until
wilted. In separate hot frying pan, place tofu with a couple of
tablespoons of oil and turn until brown. Mix vegetables together and put tofu on top. Pour sauce over them and serve.

SAUCE

Add cornstarch to ¼ cup cold water. Stir until dissolved. In a small pot, boil remaining water. Add soy sauce, oil, and marijuana and season to taste. When water boils, add water-cornstarch mix, stirring constantly. When it boils again, cornstarch will thicken liquid.

NON-FOOD INGESTION PREPARATIONS

CAPSULES

Eating marijuana in food to provide relief is a fine way of getting the medicine. However, it's not necessary to eat constantly to get relief. Clients of many buyers' clubs have found that marijuana capsules are a convenient way to take the herb.

Marijuana capsules are simple to make. First, at a health food store or drugstore, buy capsules of a size that is convenient for you to swallow. Then make a paste of one gram ground marijuana, a drop of lecithin, and just enough olive oil to make the paste on the dry side. Stuff the bottom part of the capsule with the paste. At the San Francisco Cultivator's Club, one gram of marijuana is stuffed into four capsules. This is convenient for the clients, who can use just a portion of the dose at a time.

Some stores and mail-order houses offer capsule stuffers, which hold the bottoms in place for easy filling and tamp them all at once.

TINCTURES

Tinctures are made by dissolving a large amount of THC in alcohol or by concentrating the solution.

For a tablespoon of tincture to equal a one-gram dose, two grams of grass are soaked in one ounce of liquor. (This has been described in the cooking section.) If the liquor is evaporated by two thirds, one teaspoon of tincture will contain the equivalent of about one gram of leaf. Alcohol-water solutions such as liquor are best concentrated by letting them evaporate in the open air or in a double boiler, in an area with good air circulation or a hood, because of the inflammability of the fumes.

MARIJUANA TINCTURE

1 pint 120-proof or stronger gin, vodka, or grain alcohol
32 grams dry weight (approximately 1⅛ oz.) whole
water-soaked leaf

Dry the marijuana in a microwave or a heated oven set low, so that you can grind it. Place in a jar with alcohol. Let soak for three days or more. Remove leaf using a coffee filter. Each tablespoon of tincture is equal to approximately a one-gram portion.

For a more concentrated solution, leave the tincture in the open air. The alcohol and some of the water will evaporate.

7

PRESCRIPTION AND PURCHASE OF MARIJUANA

DOONESBURY
by Garry Trudeau

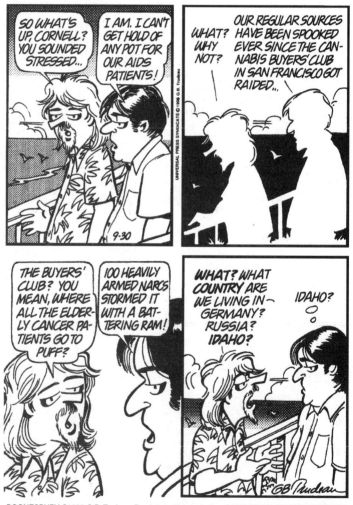

7

PRESCRIPTION AND PURCHASE OF MARIJUANA

It is illegal in the U.S. for a doctor to prescribe marijuana, because it is listed as a Schedule 1 drug. This means that the government considers the drug to have no medicinal value. Doctors sometimes write notes for patients, stating that they would prescribe marijuana if they were allowed to. This can help a patient who faces legal difficulties or seeks to join a buyers' club. It is strongly advisable to obtain a physician's support to protect yourself from legal prosecution.

One patient, Todd McCormick, who had operations for several childhood cancers, has imported medical marijuana into the U.S. He received a prescription in Holland and had it filled. He declared it at customs and they permitted him to carry it through.

GOVERNMENT COMPASSIONATE USE PROGRAM

The federal government runs the remnants of its small Compassionate Use program through the National Institute on Drug Abuse (NIDA). Today, only eight patients are receiving marijuana grown at the University of Mississippi. Each patient receives ten 0.8-gram joints of marijuana per day, 300 joints per month. The quality of the marijuana is terrible. Consisting of low potency (2–3% THC) leaf, it has earned the nickname "Mississippi ditchweed." President Bush felt that this program set a bad example and inspired hopes of a rational policy, so it

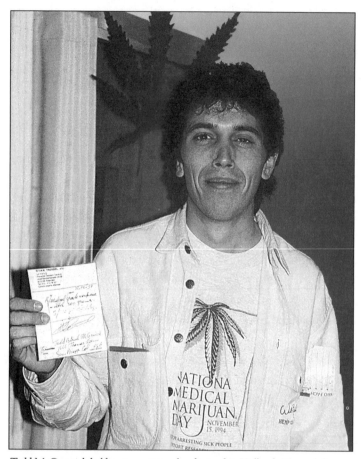

Todd McCormick holding prescription he obtained in Holland. He used the prescription to pass through customs when bringing back marijuana in 1995.

was ended in 1988. The government's reason was that it "sent the wrong message."

No state currently runs programs providing marijuana. Over 30 states have tried to enact some kind of medical marijuana research program, only to be blocked by the federal government.

However, the same Todd McCormick who brought in his medical prescription marijuana was driving cross-country when his vehicle was stopped and 31 pounds of marijuana were discovered. It was destined for the Rhode Island Medical Marijuana Buyers' Club. Eventually the judge threw out the case and ordered the medicine returned. This saga is still unfolding as we go to press.

PURCHASE

Since medical avenues are closed, patients must purchase their marijuana surreptitiously. This can be a simple transaction or a dangerous excursion, depending on the circumstances. Whatever the situation, we advise you to pay attention to your intuition and attempt to purchase only in a comfortable situation.

WHERE TO FIND MARIJUANA
CANNABIS BUYERS' CLUBS

Cannabis Buyers' Clubs for medical patients are now active in a growing number of communities: San Francisco, Los Angeles,

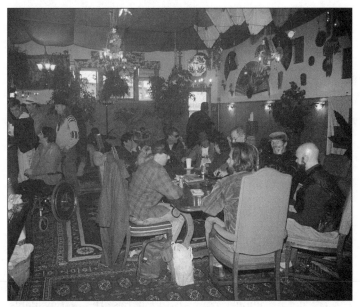

San Francisco Cultivator's Club.

New York, Seattle, and Boston to name just a few. These are probably the safest places to buy marijuana. They offer a supportive environment and a selection of different types and grades of marijuana. Some of the clubs also serve as social clubs. For you to join, most clubs require either medical records or a recommendation from your doctor. Since it is illegal for doctors to prescribe marijuana, as we have explained, some doctors write a note stating, "Marijuana would be beneficial for this condition," or "If I were allowed to, I would prescribe marijuana for this patient."

YOUR CHILDREN, GRANDCHILDREN, OR OTHER RELATIVES

You may have a relative who you know uses marijuana. Perhaps a sibling, parent, child, grandchild, or cousin will be able to obtain marijuana for your medical needs.

FRIENDS

People you know who use marijuana can purchase for you, or introduce you to their dealers.

DEALERS

Finding a dealer without an intermediary to introduce you can be very difficult. Since there are severe criminal penalties for marijuana sales, dealers are wary of making contacts without recommendations. A good dealer does not search for customers. S/he builds up a clientele of repeat buyers, usually friends of customers, and business keeps getting better—safely.

Dealers are very much like greengrocers. Since there is no standard product, the retailer's eye and taste buds determine what is stocked. The quality of fresh produce varies from store to store, as does the price. Dealers function in the same type of environment. They buy buds from wholesalers and sell retail. A good dealer has enough contacts to purchase the best available at the price, which is mostly dependent on quality, but also reflects how close the dealer is to the original source, the quantity s/he turns over, and the season.

Honest sellers of high-quality merchandise rarely have complaints from their customers, even if their prices are high. Just as in other transactions, customers' two major complaints are low quality and short weight. Dealers who sell less weight than they claim must constantly seek new customers, since the first transaction is usually the last.

STREET DEALERS

These dealers are the least likely to sell you quality marijuana, since economically they are at the bottom of the heap. They buy tiny quantities, which they divide up into minute packages. If the local government is waging an anti-pot campaign, the "dealer" could be part of a reverse sting, in which customers are arrested.

SMUGGLING

This is not a casual activity. People have fewer rights at the border than anywhere else. Unless a person knows what s/he is doing, smuggling can have disastrous results.

The reason smuggling is so tempting is that the U.S. has two long and rather porous borders. Thousands of cars cross our borders with both Canada and Mexico every day.

In Mexico, marijuana sells for between one third and one fifth the U.S. price. Western Canadian prices have dropped as a result of the northern government's harm reduction (as opposed to "lock-'em-up") policies. Indoor production of sinsemilla has increased dramatically and British Columbia has started exporting to the U.S. Prices there are one third to two thirds those in the U.S.

8

GROWING YOUR OWN

DOONESBURY
by Garry Trudeau

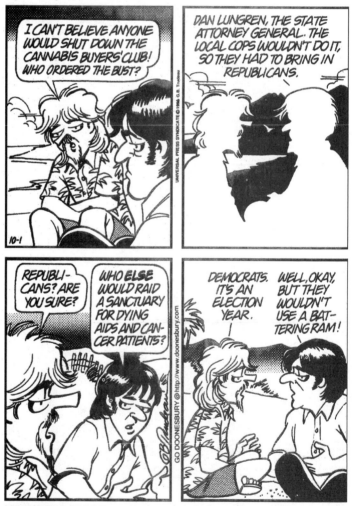

8

GROWING YOUR OWN

Although using marijuana is not addictive, growing marijuana may very well be. Aside from the many wonderful medical and psychological effects of the herb, the plant itself has many very pleasant qualities. It's easy to take care of, fast-growing, adaptable, and individualistic; it responds to its environment very quickly and very noticeably.

Marijuana's whole life cycle, from germination to ripening buds, takes only a few months, so a garden is not necessarily a long-term commitment. More important, a garden will produce usable material in a couple of months.

GROWING INDOORS

It is by far easier and more secure to grow marijuana indoors. The plants grow in the privacy of your home, safe from the eyes of others. Growing under controlled conditions has other advantages, too. The plants can be grown all year 'round and forced to flower any time you want, and they're safe from predators and from most pests.

To grow and yield buds, plants need a suitable growing environment for their tops and roots, light, good air, and certain nutrients.

Although marijuana can be grown in shorter spaces, the minimum height for comfortable growing is 5 feet. Even that limits your options, but you will be able to grow a fine crop in that space. Gardens smaller than that have special requirements, which are more thoroughly discussed in two books, *The Closet Cultivator's Guide* and *The Marijuana Grower's Handbook*.

Your space should have an adequate source of ventilation so that air, heat, and moisture can be circulated and exchanged. A natural place for the plants would be a southern window that gets exposure all day. Unfortunately, though, because of the laws, using windows is out of the question. One grower solved this problem by using skylights. He gets the sun all day without any risk of detection.

Because the plants must be hidden, most indoor gardeners use a closet, a spare room, or another discreet space. The plants are grown under lights; reflective material is used to make sure most of the light reaches the garden.

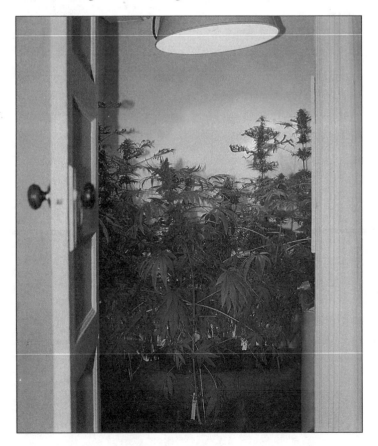

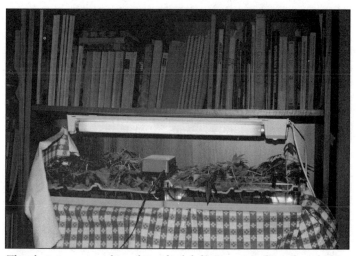

This cloning setup was located in a bookshelf. For camouflage, the cultivator used a curtain and then pinned a cardboard-backed poster to the shelves.

The plants need adequate air circulation to keep the temperature down. This can be a problem because of the electrical lighting. Also, CO_2, which is used by plants for photosynthesis, must be replaced using either fresh air or, more efficiently, a CO_2 tank and regulator.

There are many choices for your planting medium. Some gardeners choose soil or potting mix, often premixed with organic fertilizers. Others use either homemade or commercial hydroponic systems.

The most efficient lights to use are metal halides (MH) or high-pressure sodium (HPS) lights. These lamps are similar to the ones used for street lighting. The MH lamps emit a white light; the HPS, the familiar orange-pink light you see in city streets. HPS lamps emit about one sixth more light than MH lamps. Both come with a ballast (transformer) and cost from $150 to $350 for a unit. Although this is a high initial outlay, these lamps are so efficient at converting electricity to light that they pay for themselves in less than a year.

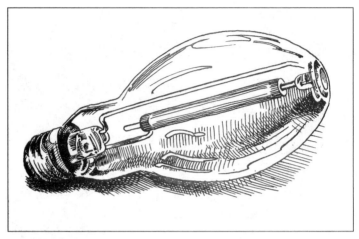

Metal Halide Lamp

Fluorescent lamps are another possibility. These tubes can be used to produce good buds, but they do have several problems. They are bulky and emit light over a large area, so it's hard to get light that's as bright as the plants need for their best growth. Also, they have only about half the efficiency of MH or HPS lamps, which means that they emit only half the light of such lamps. Fluorescent lamps do have some advantages, though. Because they emit light over a wide area, no part of the tube is too bright to come close to the plants, so they can be used in innovative ways in the garden.

Fluorescent tubes are coated with phosphors to make them emit different spectrums of light. The terms "cool white," "warm white," and "daylight" refer to these spectrums. The best combination of tubes for indoor gardens is one incandescent fluorescent, two deluxe warm white, and one cool white. The incandescent fluorescent is a fluorescent that emits the same spectrum as an incandescent (screw-in) bulb.

For fast growth, most varieties of cannabis require about 20 watts of MH or HPS, or 30 watts of fluorescent light, per square foot of garden space during the vegetative cycle.

For a good yield of buds—the part of the plant that you're trying to produce—the garden should be given 30 to 50 watts per square foot from HPS or from a mixture of HPS and MH lamps. If possible, fluorescent-lit gardens should be given 40 to 60 watts per square foot.

Incandescent "grow bulbs" are not a good way to grow plants. Although they're inexpensive to purchase, they're really more expensive than MH or HPS lamps once the cost of elec-

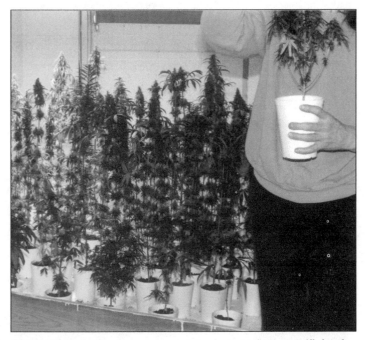

These single stem plants were grown in 32-ounce styrofoam cups filled with a mixture of vermiculite and perlite. The cups were placed in a kiddie pool to prevent spills. They were watered daily with a dilute nitrient water solution. The plants were started from cuttings and when they reached one foot they were forced to flower.

tricity is figured in. They emit only one sixth the light per unit of electricity, so the total cost for the lamp plus the electricity is higher than that for any other fixture.

There are many different ways to grow marijuana and they cannot all be covered here. Instead, we will go into just a few of the easiest methods.*

When most people imagine a marijuana plant, they see a tall, Christmas-tree-shaped bush. This image hardly matches the reality. Marijuana grown indoors is usually forced to flower when it is between 12 and 24 inches. At maturity, the plants are only 2 to 3 feet tall. Instead of a breadth of 3 or 4 feet, they are spaced at between four per square foot and one every 2 square feet. This is why they are grown in containers of different sizes and gardeners employ many different techniques to care for them. Here are just a few.

Some gardeners prefer growing in soil or potting mix. Marijuana does best in a nutrient-rich, well-drained medium with a pH of between 6 and 7. Others use planting mixes, which are not really soil, but a combination of plant products, such as bark and moss, often mixed with sand or processed minerals. In either case, the medium contains a limited amount of nutrients. These must be resupplied using either slow-release ingredients or fertilizers added to the mix at planting, or soluble fertilizers added to the water.

For plants growing 4 per square foot, a container about 6 inches across, which holds about 40 ounces of soil, is usually used. A plant growing in an area 2' x 2' could be grown in an 8-inch container, but will have a better yield if it is grown in a 1-gallon or, even better, a 3-gallon container.

....

* For a more extensive discussion of cultivation methods, we suggest either *Closet Cultivator's Guide* or *The Marijuana Grower's Handbook*, both published by Quick American Archives.

Plants grown in soil should be kept moist, so that the leaves never wilt from drought, but the roots should have access to plenty of air, so the soil cannot be kept soggy.

Indoor garden stores sell hydroponic units based on different methods of irrigating plants. While these are often on the expensive side, they usually work well, are convenient to set up and use, and are a one-time investment. Many of these units work well in a small garden and may be worth the price for the effort they save the grower. They require only a small space to support even large plants and are very clean, since no soil or potting mix is used.

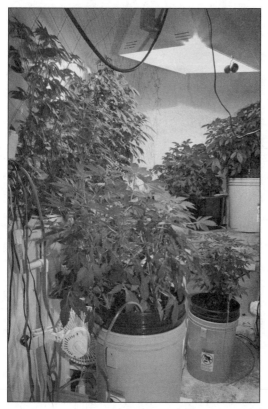

Larger plants are usually grown in commercial recirculating hydroponic units. The recirculating system is powered by inexpensive fish tank air pumps. The plants to the left are tied to a screen to keep them close to the wall so that they don't block the light.

Two very simple hydroponic units can be made very inexpensively in less than an hour.

THE RESERVOIR METHOD

Find 2' x 2' trays or smaller trays that are at least 6 inches deep. we have seen people use dishpan and restaurant dish trays. Fill 6-inch-wide plastic garden pots with ¼- or ½-inch-size crushed lava or expanded clay pellets, or a mixture of two parts large-size perlite, one part large-size vermiculite, and one part fish tank gravel or horticultural sand. Add ½ teaspoon dolomitic lime to each container. Place the containers side by side in the trays. Put an air bubbler rod, attached to a small air pump, into the tray. Add 3 inches of water-nutrient solution to the tray and you are ready to plant or transplant.

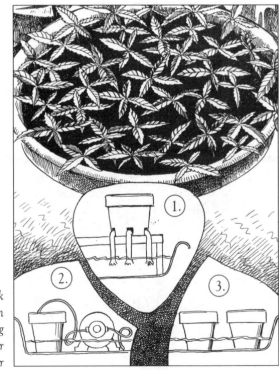

1. Wick
System
2. Recirculating
Reservoir
3. Reservoir

THE WICK MODEL

This arrangement requires the same equipment we've described above, but also some $\frac{3}{8}$" braided nylon cord and some lengths of 2" x 4" lumber, or some bricks, for the containers to rest on.

With the wick model, you have a wider choice of potting mixes. Virtually any soil, potting mix, or mix of mediums will work. One that works exceptionally well is two parts each vermiculite and perlite, and one part each aquarium gravel and either earthworm castings or humus. Add $\frac{1}{2}$ teaspoon dolomitic lime.

Place the supports in the tray. Run the cords through holes on opposite sides of the containers, with 3 inches of cord draped out from either side. Fill the containers with planting medium. Make sure the wicks drape into the tray. Then fill the trays with the water-nutrient solution. The wicks will draw up water as it is needed to keep the medium moist.

To get these systems started, water the medium until the water begins to drain from the holes. After that, you'll never need to water the individual containers; just maintain a water level in the trays. Don't add more fertilizer when you add additional water, but adjust the pH to between 6 and 7 using pH paper or a tester for measurement and raise or lower the pH to reach the right level.

These two systems produce the same results as the high-priced ones, but they have no moving parts or moving water, so it's unlikely that you'll have an accident with them.

Getting fresh air for the plants through good ventilation is important for several reasons. Bringing in new air and getting rid of the old is a good way to get rid of excess heat and moisture. Under ordinary conditions, marijuana fares best when the temperatures are in the low 70s. With enriched CO_2, the temperature should be the low 80s. A good humidity level is about 50%. The ventilation fan, which pulls out the heated and humidified air, can be regulated by a simple humidistat-thermostat.

The air in the room should be circulated too. This is because the air surrounding the leaf surface is depleted of CO_2 rather quickly. For the leaf to capture more gas, it must have a constantly renewed supply of air. Both mounted and rotating fans do this job well.

Air is constantly depleted of its CO_2 and must either be enriched or be replaced. The air should be completely replaced every six minutes. In a small closet, this can be as simple as using an open door and a fan that blows out into the room. The larger the space, the more the heat and humidity buildup, so with a larger grow room the air replacement becomes more critical. During the summer, heat may become a real problem, since the incoming air itself may be too hot for the garden. Air conditioners and air coolers can be used; you can also just shut down until the weather is more temperate.

CO_2—carbon dioxide—is an odorless, colorless gas that is not poisonous and not inflammable. It is the product of

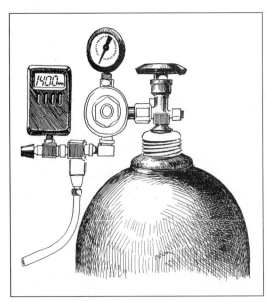

oxidation (in which oxygen combines with carbon). We breathe it out because oxidation is part of the metabolism of our bodies. In the air, it makes up about 400 parts per million (ppm) of the air.

Green plants use CO_2 during photosynthesis. It is combined with hydrogen from water to produce sugar and free
oxygen; light provides the power for the reaction. Certain
plants, including marijuana, can photosynthesize much more
quickly when the amount of CO_2 in the air is increased to
1000–1500 ppm. However, when the supply goes down to 200
ppm, they stop photosynthesizing and producing sugar, which
is what they use both for energy and as building material for
plant tissue.

Commercial nurseries supply their plants with CO_2 by burning natural gas. In the home garden, it is usually supplied by a
gas tank and regulator. The CO_2 is dispensed on the basis of
either time or measurement of the gas in the space. Although
such a setup is fairly costly, it is inexpensive to maintain and
the savings realized from it are extraordinary. Growing and
ripening time decreases by 10% to 30%; in this decreased time,
yield increases by up to 40%. Although extra CO_2 is not necessary for the garden, it makes a big difference.

Many hydroponic fertilizers suitable for growing marijuana
can be found at your local indoor garden store. They usually
come in a vegetative formula and a bloom formula. Some are
two- or three-part mixes. Each brand has its advocates and its
detractors. Their varied experiences are based in part on the
different growing methods used, the different needs of individual varieties, and the variations in water quality. We use a mix
of formulas to get the proportions we prefer. For vegetative
growth, we use something like the ratio 5-3-7 plus micronutrients; for flowering, 2-5-3 plus micronutrients. Growers have
been very successful using many different formulas; the plants
are very adaptable.

Most of the fertilizer mixes may be deficient in two essential
minerals: calcium (Ca) and magnesium (Mg). Ca is likely to be a

problem if none is listed on the fertilizer label and there are few organic ingredients in the medium or potting mix. This problem is easily solved by adding hydrated lime to the water before watering the containers, or by adding lime to the trays or reservoirs.

Mg deficiencies are solved by dissolving a teaspoon of Epsom salts ($MgSO_4$) per gallon of water once a month in soil, or every time the hydroponic water is changed.

Once the garden has been set up, it is time to plant the seeds (or transplant the rooted cuttings). The advantage of cuttings is that a cutting is known to be female. Since the males will otherwise have to be found and discarded, this eliminates a lot of effort. The quality of the individual plant is also known. Of course, the cutting should come from an outstanding plant. Since it has exactly the same genetic makeup as the plant from which it was taken, it will produce approximately the same quality and yield.

Seeds should be planted about $1/2$ inch deep. If you're using a medium such as expanded clay pellets, which will not hold the seeds securely, just add a little vermiculite at the top of the container to make a bed for the seed. The seed should germinate within a week.

If you're using either a potting mix or either of the hydroponic systems we've described, rooted cuttings are transplanted to their new containers with the rootball left intact. With some commercial systems, the directions state that the roots are placed in the system with no medium.

Plants growing in soil should be kept moist but not wet. Some growers keep the medium a little on the dry side. In any case, the containers should be watered before the soil dries or the plants show any sign of wilting.

If you're growing in soil, you should fertilize the plants with a water-soluble formula, adding it each time you water them.

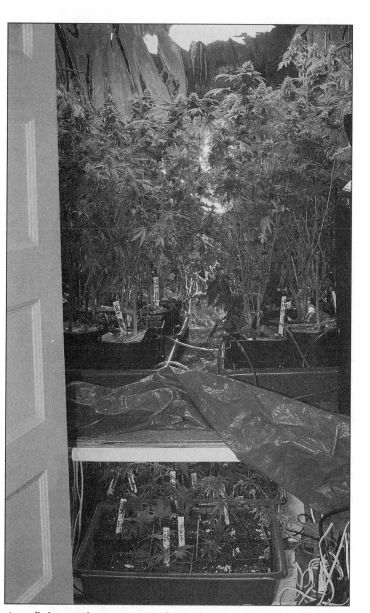

A small closet garden in a 4" x 4" closet. The clones below are in trays using Oasis rooting tubes. They are illuminated by 4" fluorescent tubes. The flowering plants, on the shelf above, are illuminated by a 400-watt HPS lamp.

Rather than using the formula at full strength once a month, as most labels recommend, it is better to supply the plants with a diluted nutrient solution each time you water them.

Once the garden has been set up, the seeds planted, and the lights and accessories turned on, most of the work is done. The seedlings or rooted cuttings begin to grow and in no time the garden is filled with greenery. If the plants are spaced close together, their leaves are probably touching and are growing on straight stems with little branching. Plants spaced farther apart usually develop more side branching, filling the space completely.

Because the plants are living in a very good environment, conducive to heavy growth, the stems may start bending or tilting a bit under the weight of the plant. Later, the heavy buds will make this even more of a problem. The solution is to use stakes or string to hold the plants upright so they don't bend over and keep the light from reaching other plants.

Once the space is filled so that there is not much light penetrating below the canopy, it is time to decide whether to just harvest leaf or go for the bud. The overwhelming majority of people prefer bud. Even if you do, you can still harvest leaf. Just clip or twist off large leaves, which interfere with light that would go to other leaves. Clipping the plant tops makes the plants "bush out" more. This practice is useful if the plants are not using the full space. It results in more, smaller buds.

If you're growing only for leaf, it's time to start harvesting. The large leaves can be removed from some plants and the tops can be cut just like a hedge. The plants will quickly regrow and can be cut again and again for many months.

When there is no longer much light penetrating below the canopy, it's also time to turn the lights down to 12 hours per day, to force the plants to flower. Remember, the plants count

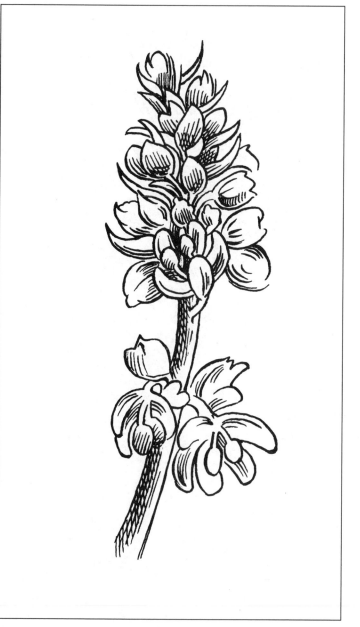

Male flower

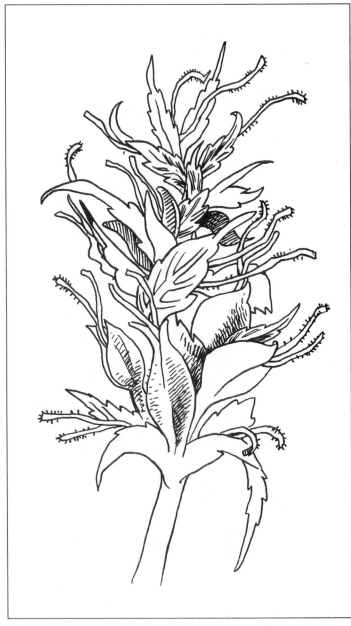

Female flower

the number of hours of uninterrupted darkness, not the number of hours of light, so it's important not to break the dark period with even the briefest moment of light.

A week after the lights are turned down, the plants' growth rate is slowed as they make the transition from vegetative to reproductive growth, which is the development of flowers. At this point, the flowers start to grow.

Unlike almost all other annual plants, each marijuana plant is either male or female. The males develop flowers first. As they are developing, the buds look something like a pawnbroker's symbol, a cluster of hanging balls. As soon as these appear, they should be removed from the garden so that they have no chance to pollinate the females. As they ripen, each little ball turns upright and opens into a tiny five-petaled flower, releasing the pollen. Pollen is very light and becomes airborne with the slightest breeze or draft.

The female flowers have no petals. Their most prominent parts are two pistils attached to a tiny ovary. At first, only a few of these flowers appear. Within weeks, thousands of them grow, filling in all the spaces so that the entire tops of the branches are thickly covered with these "hairs." Between 55 and 90 days from the time the lights were turned down, the flowers, which densely cover the stems, become ripe. The glands, which can be seen on all the leaves and vegetation surrounding the pistils, fill with the cannabinoids and look like mushrooms, a stem topped with a bulging cap. They are reaching peak potency. Another sign of ripening is that the pistils begin to dry and change color, usually to red or purple.

It is now time to harvest. This is done by cutting the stems that bear the ripe buds. Some of the lower buds may still have to ripen; these should be left on the plant. They may take another 7 to 10 days to reach maturity.

Right: Male flowers. Before the tiny five-petalled flowers open, the buds hang down from their stems looking something like a pawnbroker's balls. As soon as the males are detected they should be removed from the garden.

Below: A young female bud 15 to 25 days after forcing. The young flowers are still growing and the glands are still forming. At this stage the flowers are not very potent.

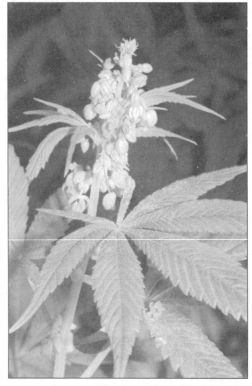

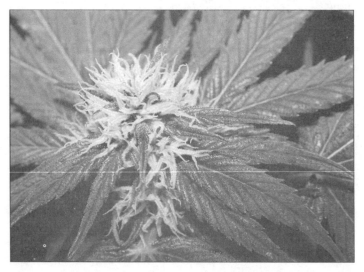

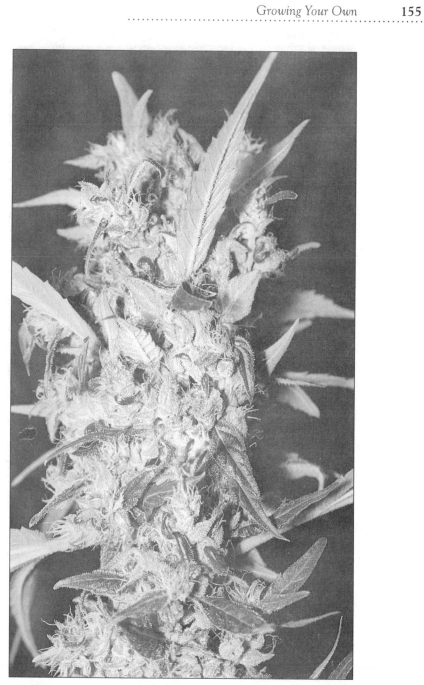

A bud about one week from harvest.

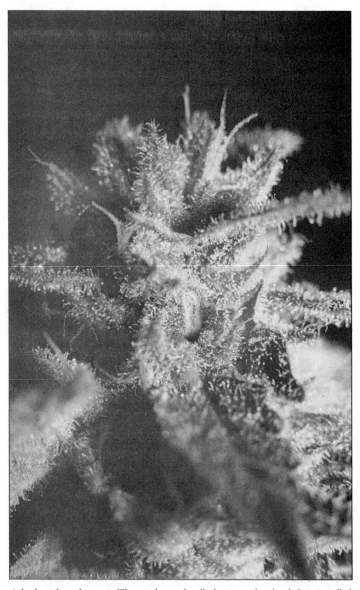

A bud ready to harvest. The pistils can hardly be seen; the glands have swelled so they shine in the light like little crystals.

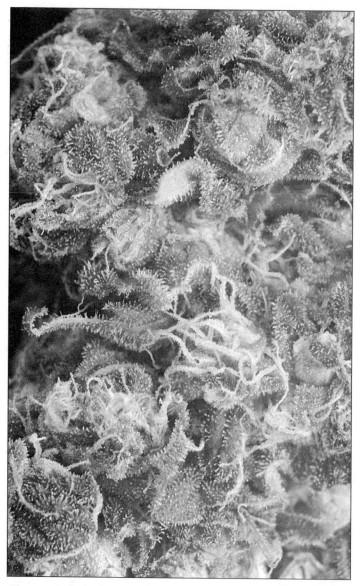

Close-up of a bud at harvest. The THC is contained in the mushroom-shaped glands covering the false seed pods.

Once the buds have been cut, they should be dried. This is best done in a cool, dark, dry place, such as a closet. The warmer and dryer it is, the faster the buds dry. Most connoisseurs find the taste mellower if the plants are dried over a 3- to 4-day period. In hot environments, buds sometimes dry in a day or less. [The buds can also be dried in a food dehydrator or microwave, but they may lose some of their odor.]

Once the buds have been harvested, there are three ways to restart the garden. These methods involve using seeds, taking cuttings, and regeneration. For most hobbyists, taking seeds and restarting is the least desirable method because of the need to separate the males, the trouble of collecting pollen from an isolated selected male, and the difficulty of pollinating selected plants.

Cuttings are an easy way to start again. A cutting produces an exact genetic duplicate of the plant it was taken from, so they are all female and can be selected from the best plants. Cuttings can be taken at any time, but those cut before any time during vegetative growth or the second week of flowering will root most easily. They should be rooted in potting medium or water, using a rooting compound, in the same way as other plant cuttings are rooted.

By far, the easiest way to restart the garden is regeneration. Keep some leaves on the plants when the buds are being harvested. Set the lights to remain on continuously for about a week and the plants will start to grow vegetatively again. Some gardeners put the plants back into harvest at this point. Others let the plants grow vegetatively for a couple more weeks and then turn the lights back down to 12 hours, which triggers flowering. One grower we know has regenerated his plants five times and is anticipating his sixth harvest.

GROWING OUTDOORS

Home growing in the U.S. started in people's backyards. A plant here and there in the garden went unnoticed until teenagers and police learned to recognize the unique shape of the marijuana leaf. Since that time, growing has gone in two different directions: indoors, under lights, and outdoors—in guerrilla gardens. [Of course, many people still do cultivate marijuana in their backyards.]

Outdoor cultivation has several advantages and several disadvantages. The main advantage is that the plant is growing in a more natural environment and nature does most of the work that you would have to do indoors. Ultimately, this means a bigger yield with less effort. Aside from the variety, the amount of sunlight, especially ultraviolet B light, that the plant receives will affect its potency. If the plants are in a mountainous, sunny spot, they will be more potent than if they grow in a shaded or cloudy area along the coast. The mountain plants may be more potent than indoor varieties.

On the other hand, growing outdoors involves environmental disadvantages. Your harvest is subject to the whims of the weather. Rain or fog during flowering promotes molds, which can ruin the crop. Unrelieved drought or extreme heat can damage or ruin a garden. Pests can devastate it in one night.

There is also the obvious element of risk. Marijuana is well recognized and, as you know, is worth money. This means that plants that are not fairly well hidden may very well be stolen. In addition, of course, there is the risk of the plants' being found out by law enforcement personnel, who may be brought to the garden by informers or by sheer chance. All this must be taken into account.

It's very easy to grow marijuana outdoors. Most varieties do best in an area that gets full sun. In places where the sun is very intense, some indoor varieties actually do better in speckled shade. The plant grows best in a nutrient-rich, well-drained soil. It is an annual, planted or transplanted at about the same time as corn or tomatoes. It can survive on a small amount of water, but to grow lushly, with a bountiful yield of buds, the plant should have ample amounts of water, about the same amount given to moderate-moisture vegetables such as corn.

During early growth, the soil is usually supplemented with a general garden formula suitable for vegetables. Starting in mid-August, the plant should be given a bloom formula, high in phosphorus (P).

As we have explained, the length of uninterrupted dark periods determines whether marijuana grows vegetatively or reproductively—whether it just continues to grow more leaves or begins to flower. Outdoors, marijuana starts to flower when the uninterrupted dark cycle reaches 10 to 12 hours, depending on the variety. Once indicas and most hybrids begin to flower, their vegetative growth slows dramatically or stops; all their energy is used to grow flowers. Sativas, which are still small because they haven't had a chance to grow, will continue to grow as they flower until they are 5 or 6 feet tall.

In the U.S., the length of the night reaches 10 hours between August 10 and September 22 in the north and July 1 and September 22 in the south. On September 22, the first day of autumn, the length of the night is 12 hours throughout the world. In some areas of the country, long-season plants do not mature before the first frost, which kills them. This is one reason why most gardeners prefer to grow indicas and hybrids rather than sativas.

Depending on the variety, the buds ripen between September and December. Indica and indica/sativa hybrids ripen from September to early November, earlier than most sativas, which originated in Mexico and Colombia. These plants are likely to ripen from mid-October through December. Seeds from domestically grown sinsemilla and near-sinsemilla may be pure indica, but they're much more likely to be hybrid.

A number of factors determine how big a marijuana plant becomes. These include the variety; growing factors including light, water, and nutrients; and the length of time the plant has been growing.

Varieties range in height from 3 to 15 feet, but most plants grow no taller than 10 feet. Indicas tend to grow smaller and more compactly, reaching only 6 to 8 feet at maturity.

Plants that are given ample amounts of light, water, and nutrients grow faster and yield more than plants that receive less. Each of these three factors is like a link of a chain: if the plant is given sufficient amounts of two of them, but not of the third, its growth is limited to the maximum amount that the third factor—the weakest link of the chain—supports.

Since marijuana's flowering is determined by the length of the uninterrupted dark cycle, plants of a single variety, even though they may be at different ages and sizes, will all flower at the same time. If there were three plants of the same variety in the garden—one transplanted in May, one in June, and one in July—they would all flower and ripen at approximately the same time. They would all be different sizes, though. Of course, the oldest plant, which had spent more time in vegetative growth, would be the largest and the youngest plant the smallest.

The home gardener growing plants in a sunny yard can expect a yield of about half an ounce per square foot of area covered by the plant's canopy. Remember, plants don't grow in rectangles, but symmetrically in circles, so the formula for plant area is pi (3.14) times the square of the radius of the plant. This is a much more significant factor than the height of the plant in determining bud yield.

Marijuana seeds can be planted directly in the soil, about $\frac{1}{2}$ inch deep, after the ground temperature reaches 70 degrees. They should be kept moist. Germination occurs within a week. Many growers start seeds indoors and then transplant the seedlings outdoors. The best, most reliable method is to use rooted cuttings from high-quality females.

CAMOUFLAGE

Marijuana is often grown with other plants in a vegetable garden, flower garden, or other planting area so that it is less easily seen. If the plant is to be trimmed back, this should be done no later than early August, so the branches have enough time to regrow and support bud growth.

Untrimmed plants grow in a symmetrical conical fashion, much like a Christmas tree. Once pruned, most varieties "bush out." Bushy plants produce more buds but smaller ones. Their total weight is often actually more than that of unpruned plants.

Plants can be tied down or manipulated into shapes that will deceive the eye. One gardener used twist-ties to attach paper flowers to her plants. Another gardener neatly trimmed parts of the characteristic "fingers" off every leaf of his plants. They looked nothing like marijuana. Another grower had morning glories climbing on his plants; their flowers covered the plants, protecting them from suspicion.

IN A YARD

As we have said, growing marijuana in your yard is a risky business. The two main pests for marijuana, both human, are thieves and the police. Both go to extraordinary lengths to find the plant. This problem is covered well in other books, so we won't go into it here.*

. . . .

* *Marijuana, the Law and You*, published by Quick American Archives covers this issue extensively.

An urban gardener had several plants, each in its own container. She started the plants in March and started to bring them outdoors in April, wheeling them out in a small cart. At night, she placed them in a dark room, making sure they got no more than 12 hours of light per day. They started to flower and were ripe in June. She kept the plants going for three weeks in vegetative mode with the help of an HPS lamp, making sure they received 18 hours of light daily. Then she brought the light cycle down for her fall harvest. Another advantage to having her plants on a cart was that she could wheel the plants into the sunny section of the garden (which changes over the course of the season).

GUERRILLA FARMING

If your view of America is shaped by the TV newsmagazine shows, you may think there are thousands of large guerrilla gardens, tended by berserk survivalists with ready trigger fingers. The truth is much duller.

The two main principles of guerrilla growing are that you are much less likely to be caught if the garden is in an area not likely to be discovered and that even if the garden is discovered, it should be so inconvenient to reach that it won't be disturbed.

Although there are some urban guerrilla farmers, most of this type of cultivation takes place in remote areas that are hard to get to, requiring considerable physical strength and endurance to reach. Such gardens are beyond the scope of this book.

We have seen a number of urban guerrilla gardens. One consisted of four female plants in September. The main stems were cut to make the plants "bush out." The site was located just beyond a railroad right of way. The plants were growing on the side of a drainage ditch along a fence, along with a number of weeds that included morning glory and lamb's quarters. To a casual viewer, they would look like just another fast-growing annual weed.

We saw another garden from a local Little League baseball field. A 25-foot retaining wall separated the field from a 30-foot-wide area that sloped up to a highway. The sloped area was fenced on the highway side and landscaped with perennials. Right in the middle of the slope, among oleander, some native buckwheat, and other highway landscape plants, were 10 young marijuana plants. They had already been pruned for bushiness, were very vigorous, and looked as if they were being fertilized, so they must have been planted. They were watered courtesy of the state.

9

A PATIENT'S STORY

DOONESBURY
by Garry Trudeau

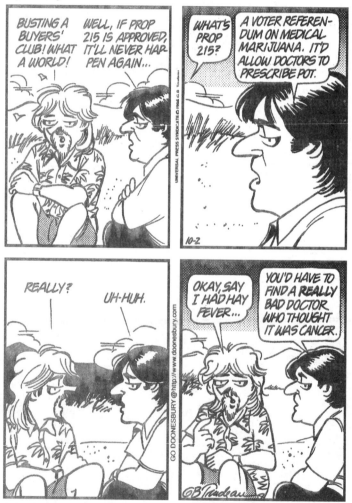

9

Medical Marijuana: A Patient's Story

I am a medical marijuana patient. For 19 years, I have grown marijuana in my vegetable and herb garden to treat my epilepsy. After some entanglement with law enforcement, I have come to realize that while patients may be protected by a specific defense of necessity, there is little to insure us against reprisals from authorities.

Medical Use

I began experimenting with marijuana after an auto accident in 1973. I suffered a closed head trauma that left me shaken by as many as five grand mal seizures per day. I became addicted to pharmaceutical medication, which nevertheless failed to relieve the seizures that plagued my life. (I am among the 25% or so of epileptics who do not respond to conventional medicines.) The prescription drugs just left me debilitated. However, I discovered that with marijuana, I could completely prevent the onset of my seizures. For me, this abilitiy meant freedom. At last I could abandon pharmaceutical medications and their side effects.

Arrest and Acquittal

In August 1992, my husband Mike and I were arrested for felony cultivation of five marijuana plants that I grow openly in our front yard. This crime is punishable by three years in state prison. After our arrest, we realized the importance of challenging the existing laws governing the medical use of marijuana. We hoped that in presenting a necessity defense we might clarify the medicinal usefulness of marijuana, freeing us from further prosecution and establishing a precedent for patients' relief.

After seven and one-half months, the district attorney of Santa Cruz County, California, dropped charges against me for marijuana cultivation. He stated, "No reasonable jury would find her guilty."

Believing I had won the right to use the only medicine that controls my seizure activity, I again planted five marijuana plants in my front garden. In September 1993, Campaign Against Marijuana Planting (CAMP) agents arrived at our home and, after a three-hour search, confiscated my medicine and arrested us.

Under ordinary circumstances, it seems that the dismissal would have set a precedent for patients who satisfy the six points of necessity for cultivation. And indeed it does. But are we protected by the law? Or are we shuffled between departments? The fact is that even though there is no alternative that will provide relief for my condition, and despite my having adequately established necessity through the judiciary system, it is still illegal, under federal law, to use or cultivate marijuana.

California State Senator Henry Mello has presented a non-binding resolution, SJR 8, in a bipartisan effort to allow the use of marijuana medicinally. There is at present no provision by the federal government to meet the needs of patients; only the remnants of the antiquated Compassionate IND (Investigational New Drug) program, currently serving eight government-approved patients, exists today. This now-defunct program supplied patients with government marijuana, but the project was axed by the Bush administration in March 1992.

RESEARCH

The Food and Drug Administration (FDA) requires three phases of study for ascertaining the acceptability of a new drug for medical use in treatment of patients. These are Phase I, safety; Phase II, pilot studies on efficacy; and Phase III, controlled studies on safety and efficacy. According to Judge Francis L. Young, presiding Administrative Law Judge to the United States Department of Justice in the DEA hearings on the Marijuana Rescheduling Petition in 1988, it has been established that marijuana satisfies Phase I, II, and Phase III studies on safety and efficacy.

Now that sufficient evidence has substantiated these findings, it seems redundant to continue further studies on the safety or efficacy of marijuana. By giving in to the FDA's present acceptance of only Phase II (safety) studies, we surrender ground we have already gained. In fact, since patients' needs are ever growing, it is essential to focus on the third phase, controlled trials, if any aspect of further research is considered necessary. To move backward into pilot research, and to focus on only that, clearly ignores the results of nearly 20 years of legal battles. Delay only creates further suffering for patients. It is urgent to create a solution to this problem and immediately meet the needs of those who are now suffering and dying.

HELPING CANCER PATIENTS

In 1978, someone I loved became ill. The diagnosis was terminal cancer in the advanced stages of leukemia. I thought marijuana might help and I encouraged her to try it, hoping it would curb her severe reaction to chemotherapy. We found that a tea solution made from marijuana reduced her nausea and helped her to sleep. She remarked, "It's the best sleep I can remember having in years." She found that her last months of life were improved by using marijuana. In 15 years, more than 20 of our friends and family members have died. Most of them have used marijuana at some time during their dying process.

Since our initial arrest, I have been inundated with calls from patients seeking protection, information, and help. I've begun working closely with terminal patients who use marijuana. From them, I have been able to collect information to begin an anecdotal efficacy study in the form of a visual analog. I will explain this visual analog in the discussion that follows.

While this type of study could conceivably track the results of marijuana use for any number of different ailments, I originally restricted my study to terminal patients. However, as an overwhelming interest grows, I have begun to offer the daily visual analog for use by certain other patients. I hope to collect a broad database to substantiate the effectiveness of marijuana on many ailments.

Any patient who meets the six points of medical necessity* would be a likely candidate for such a study. I have encountered no objection to the use of marijuana by the medical profession in cases of AIDS, cancer, glaucoma, and my own case of epilepsy.

I was contacted by H. A., a terminal patient who has pancreatic and liver cancer. We discussed how we might develop a simple record of his marijuana use in order to register its effects on his dying process. Together, we were able to expand a general daily visual analog to collect data from patients who use marijuana. It features a graph on which a patient can record

----

* The Six Points of Medical Necessity are:
The act charged as a crime must have been done to prevent a significant evil; the harm caused by the act must not be disproportionate to the harm avoided; the accused must entertain a good faith belief that the act was necessary to prevent greater harm; the belief must be objectively reasonable under all of the circumstances; there is no adequate alternative to the commission of the act, and the accused must not have contributed to the creation of the emergency.

responses both before and after marijuana use under different categories.

In a recent conversation with H. A., we talked extensively about his illness. He has lived for a remarkable three years with his diagnosis. I asked him to tell me what marijuana did for him and why he thinks he has defied the odds of a six-month prognosis. He mentioned the usual benefits: heightened energy, increased appetite, pain relief, and so on. Then he said a most remarkable thing! He told me that marijuana changed his perception.

REDUCED PAIN AND DISTRESS

We have found that while it is apparent that marijuana can be used to help ailing patients both to sleep and to "get the munchies," it has a deep effect on pain and helps some patients achieve an altered level of awareness.

How can this altered state be of importance in the treatment of terminally ill patients? H. A. says that while he feels marijuana has prolonged his life because he enjoys a ravenous appetite, another factor is also important. He states that marijuana alters the way he perceives his inevitable death. He insists that his marijuana use has helped him to accept his illness and its eventual outcome. His wife says that he has regained his sense of humor. Not many of us can smile in the face of such a reality.

Working with H. A. has opened my mind to a great hidden issue that lies at the heart of considerations of this plant medicine. Why shouldn't we alter our consciousness? Of the many terminal patients to whom I have had the opportunity to provide some assistance, I have seen time and again that although there is often little we can do to alter a situation, we can change our view of it. For some people, marijuana can do this.

One of the major causes of failure in any treatment for pain is the failure to differentiate pain from suffering. If a patient thinks s/he feels better when using marijuana, then what is the difference between that idea and actually feeling better?

In the first four months that I worked with H. A., he cut his extensive chronic use of the addictive drug Dilaudid and did not renew his prescription for this painkiller over a period of four months, relying solely on marijuana. Recently he ran out of marijuana and was subsequently admitted to the hospital for pain control, at a cost of $8,000. Such an example of the prohibitive cost of medical care provides a substantial reason for allowing patients to meet their own needs by growing marijuana for personal use. A few weeks later, H. A. ran out again. His doctor advised another hospital stay to control his pain. H. A. suggested an attempt to procure more marijuana. He received his medicine and stayed out of the hospital. His doctor was enthusiastic about the results.

Another terminal patient, with bone cancer, began using marijuana baked in cake and brownies at the onset of his two-week prognosis. This was nearly six weeks ago. Shortly after he began ingesting marijuana, he started a rigorous chemotherapy treatment, consisting of Cisplatin, in conjunction with other pharmaceutical drugs. He managed the first part of the week-long treatment with only one bout of nausea and he gained 6 pounds. His doctor and his hospice nurse applauded his marijuana use.

During our last visit, he told me there is no doubt in his mind that marijuana is the cause of his success. (He did suggest that the addition of a few chocolate chips to the brownies would create a near-perfect medicine.)

HELPING SPASTICITY PATIENTS

I asked a 32-year-old spinal cord injury victim what kind of alternatives were available in lieu of using marijuana for spasticity. He said he had been offered either drugs—muscle relaxants, opiates, and antidepressants—or a procedure whose preliminary therapeutic techniques include surgical alteration of muscle tissue to relieve spasticity. Certainly neither of these seems any more reasonable than simply smoking or ingesting marijuana.

A 100% disabled veteran has abandoned the use of pharmaceutical drugs, including Ativan and various pain medications, which he has relied on for over 20 years, by replacing them with marijuana brownies. This inexpensive alternative protects him from depression, anxiety, and mood swings. Marijuana affords him the opportunity to be a productive member of society and a more conscientious father. Before his marijuana use, he says, he would often lie about the house under the influence of the pharmaceuticals for days at a time. He states that replacing drugs with marijuana has improved his attitude. He adds that he is finding a way out of the depression that Ativan causes, while the pain of arthritis from a war wound has diminished and is also easier for him to accept.

PATIENT RIGHTS

As a Schedule I drug, marijuana is considered dangerous and of no medicinal value. In this light, it is difficult to understand the DEA's position on this issue when the FDA provides a marijuana derivative called Marinol to some patients. It is curious that the FDA and pharmaceutical companies pursue the development of synthetic marijuana if indeed it has no medicinal use. If the FDA and the DEA succeed, patients may come under further pressure to forfeit their ability to use this plant medicine in its natural form.

The life of a patient is restricted by illness. Being able to have a hands-on approach to relieve their suffering by growing their own medicine can be an extremely valuable and empowering experience. For many, this is a simple action they can take for themselves to provide free health care and vitally important quality control. Purity of medicine is imperative to prevent further health problems, such as those associated with molds, toxins, or chemical impurities. For instance, spergillosis, caused by mold, presents an acute pneumonia that occurs in immunosuppressed patients. High-quality, high-potency marijuana, available in many varieties, can have far-reaching effects on a wide range of symptoms of illness.

For the many patients whose diagnoses include cancer, AIDS, epilepsy, birth defects, glaucoma, and spasticity, marijuana provides answers. When a patient has no alternative to rely on for relief, it is likely that s/he meets the six points of necessity. Protection lies in establishing credible testimony to meet the six points. Substantial evidence to support such a defense must be presented. It is extremely important for a patient to notify a physician of her/his marijuana use. It's necessary to examine the six elements that constitute a necessity defense and discuss alternative medicine with the physician. Be certain that such information is entered in your medical record. Documentation is everything.

Not everyone is protected by this procedure. Though any ailment should be relieved, not every patient will be able to prove all six points. There is a question as to the existence of an "adequate alternative" to an FDA-approved drug. If an adequate alternative exists, what kind of side effects does it produce? Does it provide the desired relief? A patient can certainly help the doctor determine the answers to these queries.

Thousands experience the fear of prosecution and the pain that must be endured when this herbal remedy is not available. Patients and caregivers take the risk of using it because there is no choice. The gap widens as we consider the many illnesses for which marijuana can provide aid. In cases such as PMS, migraine headaches, depression, and any number of other debilitating maladies that may not be considered life-threatening, there seems to be a great deal of resistance to the acceptance of marijuana as treatment.

The six points of medical necessity are meant to identify a situation in which no other means of action can prevent a patient's disorder. A court might reject a defense of medical necessity if the accused were not suffering from a seriously debilitating disease.

REDUCED MEDICAL COSTS

Among the patients I've worked with, one recurring theme is the financial burden that illness brings. Even when an insurance company pays up to 80% of medical costs, paying the remainder can shatter fragile finances. I have spoken with families who have lost much of their life savings, or sold their cars and heirlooms to come up with the copayments on their hospital bills. This is quite common.

Free medical care can be augmented by providing for oneself. Marijuana is a plant that can be grown at almost no cost in a garden, in a closet, or on a patio. Assistance for those who do not garden could be provided through government or private agencies. Some patients or caregivers might choose to grow this herbal medicine and could do so with a doctor's prescription and a permit. A doctor could surely determine how to prescribe it just as s/he does with other medicines.

It's obvious that an underground exists to offer supplies of marijuana. The "war on drugs" has skyrocketed to include grandmothers with cancer and their backyard gardens, caregivers growing a few plants for loved ones, and friends helping friends by hitting the streets in search of this proven remedy. These practices have been made both risky and costly. It's expensive to be sick in America.

We are patients challenged by the drawbacks of our diseases. Our primary concern in using marijuana is not how it hinders us, but how it makes us well. Compared with the pharmacopoeia of synthetic alternatives that many of us have been offered, this natural medicine enables us to function in our daily lives, and for some of us it furnishes a view that reaches far beyond our limitations.

As patients, we grope through the darkness of our illness without knowing from where relief will come. We hope that there will be an end to our suffering. When we find one, there is little that could deter us from its use or convince us of its evil.

—by Valerie Corral

APPENDICES

Appendix 1

CALIFORNIA BUYERS' CLUBS

Hayward
Hayward Cannabis Buyer's Club
P.O. Box 22540, Main Street, Box 333, Hayward, CA 94541
Tel. 510-330-7333

Los Angeles
West Hollywood, Tel. 213-874-0811

Marin
Marin Alliance for Medical Marijuana
Tel. 415-256-9328

Oakland
Oakland Cannabis Buyer's Co-op
P.O. Box 24590, Oakland, CA 94623
Tel. 510-832-5346, Fax 510-986-0534

Sacramento
Capitol City Cannabis Buyer's Club
P.O. Box 188056, Sacramento, CA 95814
Tel. 916-448-6442

San Francisco
Cannabis Helping Alleviate Medicinal Problems (CHAMP)
194 Church Street, San Francisco, CA 94114
Tel. 415-861-1040, Fax 415-861-1001

Flower Therapy
3180 17th Street, San Francisco, CA 94110
Tel. 415-255-6305, Fax 415-255-6305

San Francisco Cultivator's Club
1444 Market Street, San Francisco, CA 94102
Tel. 415-621-3986

Santa Cruz
Wo-Men's Alliance for Medical Marijuana
(Special Services Distribution)
Santa Cruz, Tel. 408-423-5413

Santa Cruz Cannabis Buyers Club
201 Maple Street, Santa Cruz, CA 95060, Tel. 408-429-8819

Appendix 2

PROPOSITION 200
ANALYSIS BY LEGISLATIVE COUNCIL
(In compliance with A.R.S. section 19-124)

Proposition 200 would require that certain persons who are convicted of drug offenses be sentenced as follows:

1. Require that persons who commit violent crimes while under the influence of drugs serve 100% of their sentences, without eligibility for parole.

2. Require that persons who have been convicted before the proposition passes of the personal possession or use of a controlled substance such as marijuana and who are serving their sentence in prison be released on parole. A person is released on parole after serving time in jail or prison, is under the supervision of a parole officer and may have his parole revoked if any condition of parole is violated. The State Department of Corrections would be required to establish a procedure for paroling these persons. The Board of Executive Clemency would be required to release these persons unless the Board determines that a person would be a danger to the general public. Persons who are released on parole would be required to participate in drug treatment or education.

3. Require that persons who are convicted after the proposition passes of the personal possession or use of a controlled substance such as marijuana be eligible for probation. A person who is sentenced to probation does not serve any time in jail or prison, is under the supervision of a probation officer and remains free as long as the person continues his good behavior. A person on probation would be required to participate in a drug treatment or education program.

Proposition 200 would allow medical doctors to prescribe a controlled substance such as marijuana to treat a disease or to relieve the pain and suffering of a seriously or terminally ill patient. The doctor must be able to document that scientific research supports the use of the controlled substance and must obtain a written opinion from a second doctor that prescribing the controlled substance is appropriate. A patient who receives, possesses or uses a controlled substance as prescribed by a doctor would not be subject to criminal penalties.

Proposition 200 would establish the Drug Treatment and Education Fund. These monies would come from a percentage of the luxury tax on alcohol, cigarettes and other tobacco products. 50% of these monies would be transferred to Superior Court probation departments to cover the costs of placing persons in drug education and treatment programs. The remaining 50% of the monies would be transferred to the Arizona Parents Commission on Drug Education and Prevention.

Proposition 200 would establish an Arizona Parents Commission on Drug Education and Prevention. The Commission would be responsible for funding programs that increase and enhance parental involvement in drug education and treatment.

PROPOSITION 200
DRUG MEDICALIZATION, PREVENTION, AND CONTROL ACT
OF 1996 — AN INITIATIVE MEASURE

AMENDING TITLE 13, TITLE 41, AND TITLE 42, OF THE ARIZONA REVISED STATUTES; AMENDING TITLE 41, CHAPTER 11, BY ADDING §41-1604.16; RELATING TO ESTABLISHMENT OF THE ARIZONA PARENTS COMMISSION ON DRUG EDUCATION AND PREVENTION; AMENDING TITLE 41, CHAPTER 11, BY ADDING §41-1604.14; RELATING TO PERSONS NOT ELIGIBLE FOR PAROLE; AMENDING TITLE 13, CHAPTER 13, BY AMENDING §13-3412 AND ADDING §13-3412.01; RELATING TO PERMISSIBLE USE OF CONTROLLED SUBSTANCES BY SERIOUSLY ILL OR TERMINALLY ILL PATIENTS; AMENDING TITLE 41, CHAPTER 11, BY ADDING §41-1604.15 AND AMENDING TITLE 31, CHAPTER 3, BY ADDING §31-411.01; RELATING TO PAROLE FOR PERSONS CONVICTED OF PERSONAL POSSESSION OR USE OF CONTROLLED SUBSTANCES; AMENDING TITLE 13, CHAPTER 9, BY ADDING §13-901.01; RELATING TO PROBATION FOR PERSONS CONVICTED OF PERSONAL POSSESSION OR USE OF CONTROLLED SUBSTANCES AND BY ADDING §13-901.02; RELATING TO THE ESTABLISHMENT OF THE DRUG TREATMENT AND EDUCATION FUND; AND AMENDING TITLE 42, CHAPTER 12, BY ADDING §42-1204.01; RELATING TO LUXURY PRIVILEGE TAXES; AND PROVIDING FOR SEVERABILITY.

TEXT OF PROPOSED AMENDMENT

Be it enacted by the people of the State of Arizona: The following amendments are proposed to become valid when approved by a majority of the qualified electors voting thereon and upon proclamation pursuant thereto by the Governor of the State of Arizona.

Section 1. TITLE

THIS ACT SHALL BE KNOWN AND MAY BE CITED AS THE "DRUG MEDICALIZATION, PREVENTION, AND CONTROL ACT OF 1996."

Section 2. FINDINGS AND DECLARATIONS

THE PEOPLE OF THE STATE OF ARIZONA FIND AND DECLARE THE FOLLOWING:

1.ARIZONA'S CURRENT APPROACH TO DRUG CONTROL NEEDS TO BE STRENGTHENED. THIS IS EVIDENCED BY THE FACT THAT, ACCORDING TO THE ARIZONA CRIMINAL JUSTICE COMMISSION, BETWEEN 1991 AND 1993 MARIJUANA USE DOUBLED AMONG ELEMENTARY SCHOOL STUDENTS AND, BETWEEN 1990 AND 1993 QUADRUPLED AMONG MIDDLE-SCHOOL STUDENTS. IN ADDITION TO ACTIVELY ENFORCING OUR CRIMINAL LAWS AGAINST DRUGS, WE NEED TO MEDICALIZE ARIZONA'S DRUG CONTROL POLICY: RECOGNIZING THAT DRUG ABUSE IS A PUBLIC HEALTH PROBLEM AND TREATING ABUSE AS A DISEASE. THUS, DRUG TREATMENT AND PREVENTION MUST BE EXPANDED.

2.WE MUST ALSO TOUGHEN ARIZONA'S LAWS AGAINST VIOLENT CRIMINALS ON DRUGS. ANY PERSON WHO COMMITS A VIOLENT CRIME WHILE UNDER THE INFLUENCE OF ILLEGAL DRUGS SHOULD SERVE 100% OF HIS OR HER SENTENCE WITH ABSOLUTELY NO EARLY RELEASE.

3.THOUSANDS OF ARIZONANS SUFFER FROM DEBILITATING DISEASES SUCH AS GLAUCOMA, MULTIPLE SCLEROSIS, CANCER, AND AIDS, BUT CANNOT HAVE ACCESS TO THE NECESSARY DRUGS THEY NEED. ALLOWING DOCTORS TO PRESCRIBE SCHEDULE I CONTROLLED SUBSTANCES COULD SAVE VICTIMS OF THESE DISEASES FROM LOSS OF SIGHT, LOSS OF PHYSICAL CAPACITY, AND GREATLY REDUCE THE PAIN AND SUFFERING OF THE SERIOUSLY ILL AND TERMINALLY ILL.

4.THE DRUG PROBLEMS OF NON-VIOLENT PERSONS WHO ARE CONVICTED OF PERSONAL POSSESSION OR USE OF DRUGS ARE BEST HANDLED THROUGH COURT-SUPERVISED DRUG TREATMENT AND EDUCATION PROGRAMS. THESE PROGRAMS ARE MORE EFFECTIVE

THAN LOCKING NON-VIOLENT OFFENDERS UP IN A COSTLY PRISON. PILOT PROGRAMS IN ARIZONA THAT PROVIDE TREATMENT ALTER-NATIVES TO PRISON FOR LOW LEVEL DRUG OFFENDERS HAVE A 73% SUCCESS RATE AND COST ROUGHLY 1/8 AS MUCH AS PRISON. OVER THE NEXT DECADE HUNDREDS OF MILLIONS OF DOLLARS CAN BE SAVED BY USING MANDATORY DRUG TREATMENT AND EDUCATION PROGRAMS AS AN ALTERNATIVE TO PRISON.

5.VIOLENT OFFENDERS ARE NOT ADEQUATELY PUNISHED DUE TO THE PRISON OVER-CROWDING CRISIS IN ARIZONA. PLACING NON-VIOLENT PERSONS WHO ARE CONVICTED OF PERSONAL POSSES-SION OR USE OF DRUGS IN COURT-SUPERVISED DRUG TREATMENT AND EDUCATION PROGRAMS WILL FREE UP SPACE IN OUR PRISONS SO THAT THERE IS ROOM TO INCARCERATE VIOLENT OFFENDERS AND DRUG DEALERS.

6.THE MISSING LINK IN DRUG EDUCATION AND PREVENTION IS PARENTAL INVOLVEMENT. THE TAX DOLLARS SAVED BY ELIMINAT-ING PRISON TIME FOR NON-VIOLENT PERSONS CONVICTED OF PER-SONAL POSSESSION OR USE OF DRUGS SHOULD BE USED FOR DRUG TREATMENT AND EDUCATION, TARGETED AT PROGRAMS THAT INCREASE PARENTAL INVOLVEMENT IN THEIR CHILDREN'S DRUG-EDUCATION.

Section 3. PURPOSE AND INTENT

THE PEOPLE OF THE STATE OF ARIZONA DECLARE THEIR PURPOSES TO BE AS FOLLOWS:

1.TO REQUIRE THAT ANY PERSON WHO COMMITS A VIOLENT CRIME UNDER THE INFLUENCE OF DRUGS SERVE 100 PERCENT OF HIS OR HER SENTENCE AND NOT BE ELIGIBLE FOR PAROLE OR ANY FORM OF EARLY RELEASE.

2.TO PERMIT DOCTORS TO PRESCRIBE SCHEDULE I CONTROLLED SUBSTANCES TO TREAT A DISEASE, OR TO RELIEVE THE PAIN AND SUFFERING OF SERIOUSLY ILL AND TERMINALLY ILL PATIENTS.

3.TO REQUIRE THAT NON-VIOLENT PERSONS CONVICTED OF PER-SONAL POSSESSION OR USE OF DRUGS SUCCESSFULLY UNDERGO COURT-SUPERVISED MANDATORY DRUG TREATMENT PROGRAMS AND PROBATION.

4.TO REQUIRE THAT NON-VIOLENT PERSONS CURRENTLY IN PRISON FOR PERSONAL POSSESSION OR USE OF ILLEGAL DRUGS, AND NOT SERVING A CONCURRENT SENTENCE FOR ANOTHER CRIME, OR PRE-VIOUSLY CONVICTED OR SENTENCED OR SUBJECT TO SENTENCING UNDER ANY HABITUAL CRIMINAL STATUTE IN ANY JURISDICTION IN THE UNITED STATES, BE MADE ELIGIBLE FOR IMMEDIATE PAROLE AND DRUG TREATMENT, EDUCATION AND COMMUNITY SERVICE.

5.TO FREE UP SPACE IN OUR PRISONS TO PROVIDE ROOM FOR VIO-LENT OFFENDERS.

6.TO EXPAND THE SUCCESS OF PILOT DRUG INTERVENTION PRO-GRAMS WHICH DIVERT DRUG OFFENDERS FROM PRISON TO DRUG TREATMENT, EDUCATION, AND COUNSELING.

Section 4.

Title 41, Chapter 11, Arizona Revised Statutes, is amended by adding §41-1604.16 to read as follows:

§41-1604.16. ARIZONA PARENTS COMMISSION ON DRUG EDUCATION AND PREVENTION.

1.THE ARIZONA PARENTS COMMISSION ON DRUG EDUCATION AND PREVENTION IS HEREBY CREATED. THE COMMISSION SHALL CON-SIST OF NINE (9) MEMBERS. THE MEMBERS OF THE COMMISSION SHALL BE APPOINTED BY THE GOVERNOR WITHIN SIXTY (60) DAYS OF THE EFFECTIVE DATE OF THIS ACT AND SHALL SERVE A TWO YEAR TERM. OF THE NINE MEMBERS, FIVE SHALL BE PARENTS WITH CHILDREN CURRENTLY ENROLLED IN AN ARIZONA SCHOOL, ONE SHALL BE A REPRESENTATIVE OF A LAW ENFORCEMENT AGENCY, ONE SHALL BE AN EDUCATOR IN A LOCAL SCHOOL DISTRICT, ONE

SHALL BE A REPRESENTATIVE OF A COUNTY PROBATION DEPART-
MENT, AND ONE SHALL BE A REPRESENTATIVE OF THE DRUG EDU-
CATION AND TREATMENT COMMUNITY.

2.EACH MEMBER SHALL BE APPOINTED FOR A TERM OF TWO YEARS.
THE MEMBERS SHALL RECEIVE NO PAY, BUT MAY BE REIMBURSED
FOR ACTUAL EXPENSES INCURRED ON COMMISSION BUSINESS.

3.THE COMMISSION SHALL FUND PROGRAMS THAT WILL INCREASE
AND ENHANCE PARENTAL INVOLVEMENT AND WILL INCREASE EDU-
CATION ABOUT THE SERIOUS RISKS AND PUBLIC HEALTH PROBLEMS
CAUSED BY THE ABUSE OF ALCOHOL AND CONTROLLED SUB-
STANCES.

4.THE COMMISSION SHALL CONTRACT FOR ADMINISTRATIVE AND
PROFESSIONAL SERVICES WITH A NOT FOR PROFIT ORGANIZATION
OR GOVERNMENT ENTITY WITH EXPERTISE IN SUBSTANCE ABUSE
EDUCATION AND PREVENTION.

Section 5.

Title 41, Chapter 11, Arizona Revised Statutes, is amended by adding §41-1604.14
to read as follows:

§41-1604.14. PAROLE NONELIGIBILITY; VIOLENT CRIME; INFLUENCE OF
CONTROLLED SUBSTANCE;

DEFINITION

1.NOTWITHSTANDING ANY LAW TO THE CONTRARY, ANY PERSON
CONVICTED OF A VIOLENT CRIME COMMITTED WHILE UNDER THE
INFLUENCE OF A CONTROLLED SUBSTANCE IN VIOLATION OF THE
PROVISIONS TITLE 13, CHAPTER 34, IS NONELIGIBLE FOR PAROLE
AND MUST SERVE 100 PERCENT OF HIS OR HER SENTENCE IN PRISON.
PURSUANT TO §41-1604.09, THE DIRECTOR SHALL INCLUDE ANY
SUCH PERSON IN THE CLASSES OF NON-ELIGIBILITY REQUIRED TO
BE ESTABLISHED BY THE DIRECTOR.

2.FOR THE PURPOSE OF THIS SECTION, A VIOLENT CRIME INCLUDES ANY CRIMINAL ACT WHICH RESULTS IN DEATH OR PHYSICAL INJURY OR ANY CRIMINAL USE OF WEAPONS OR DANGEROUS INSTRUMENTS.

Section 6.

Title 13, Chapter 13, §13-3412, Arizona Revised Statutes, is amended as follows:

§13-3412. Exceptions and exemptions; burden of proof; privileged communications.

1.The provisions of §§13-3402, 13-3403, 13-3404, 13-3404.01 and 13-3405 through 13-3409 do not apply to:

1.Manufacturers, wholesalers, pharmacies and pharmacists under the provisions of §32-1921 and 32-1961.

2.Medical practitioners, pharmacies and pharmacists while acting in the course of their professional practice, in good faith and in accordance with generally accepted medical standards.

3.Persons who lawfully acquire and use such drugs only for scientific purposes.

4.Officers and employees of the United States, this state or a political subdivision of the United States or this state, while acting in the course of their official duties.

5.An employee or agent of a person described in paragraphs 1 through 4 of this subsection, and a registered nurse or medical technician under the supervision of a medical practitioner, while such employee, agent, nurse or technician is acting in the course of professional practice or employment, and not on his own account.

6.A common or contract carrier or warehouseman, or an employee of such carrier or warehouseman, whose possession of such drugs is in the usual course of business or employment.

7.Persons lawfully in possession or control of controlled substances authorized by title 36, chapter 27.

8.Persons who sell any non-narcotic substance that under the federal food, drug and cosmetic act may lawfully be sold over the counter without a prescription.

9.THE RECEIPT, POSSESSION OR USE, OF A CONTROLLED SUBSTANCE INCLUDED IN SCHEDULE I OF §36-2512, BY ANY SERIOUSLY ILL OR TERMINALLY ILL PATIENT, PURSUANT TO THE PRESCRIPTION OF A DOCTOR IN COMPLIANCE WITH THE PROVISIONS OF §13-3412.01.

2.In any complaint, information or indictment and in any action or proceeding brought for the enforcement of any provision of this chapter the burden of proof of any such exception, excuse, defense or exemption is on the defendant.

3.In addition to other exceptions to the physician-patient privilege, information communicated to a physician in an effort to procure unlawfully a prescription-only, dangerous or narcotic drug, or to procure unlawfully the administration of such drug, is not a privileged communication.

Section 7.

Title 13, Chapter 13, Arizona Revised Statutes, is amended by adding §13-3412.01 to read as follows:

§13-3412.01. PRESCRIBING CONTROLLED SUBSTANCES INCLUDED IN SCHEDULE I OF §36-2512 FOR SERIOUSLY ILL AND TERMINALLY ILL PATIENTS

1.NOTWITHSTANDING ANY LAW TO THE CONTRARY, ANY MEDICAL DOCTOR LICENSED TO PRACTICE IN ARIZONA MAY PRESCRIBE A CONTROLLED SUBSTANCE INCLUDED IN SCHEDULE I OF §36-2512 TO TREAT A DISEASE, OR TO RELIEVE THE PAIN AND SUFFERING OF A SERIOUSLY ILL PATIENT OR TERMINALLY ILL PATIENT, SUBJECT TO THE PROVISIONS OF §13-3412.01. IN PRESCRIBING SUCH A CON-TROLLED SUBSTANCE, THE MEDICAL DOCTOR SHALL COMPLY WITH PROFESSIONAL MEDICAL STANDARDS.

2.NOTWITHSTANDING ANY LAW TO THE CONTRARY, A MEDICAL DOCTOR MUST DOCUMENT THAT SCIENTIFIC RESEARCH EXISTS WHICH SUPPORTS THE USE OF A CONTROLLED SUBSTANCE LISTED IN SCHEDULE I OF §36-2512 TO TREAT A DISEASE, OR TO RELIEVE THE PAIN AND SUFFERING OF A SERIOUSLY ILL PATIENT OR TERMINALLY ILL PATIENT BEFORE PRESCRIBING THE CONTROLLED SUBSTANCE. A

MEDICAL DOCTOR PRESCRIBING A CONTROLLED SUBSTANCE INCLUDED IN SCHEDULE I OF §36-2512 TO TREAT A DISEASE, OR TO RELIEVE THE PAIN AND SUFFERING OF A SERIOUSLY ILL PATIENT OR TERMINALLY ILL PATIENT, MUST OBTAIN THE WRITTEN OPINION OF A SECOND MEDICAL DOCTOR THAT THE PRESCRIBING OF THE CONTROLLED SUBSTANCE IS APPROPRIATE TO TREAT A DISEASE OR TO RELIEVE THE PAIN AND SUFFERING OF A SERIOUSLY ILL PATIENT OR TERMINALLY ILL PATIENT. THE WRITTEN OPINION OF THE SECOND MEDICAL DOCTOR SHALL BE KEPT IN THE PATIENT'S OFFICIAL MEDICAL FILE. BEFORE PRESCRIBING THE CONTROLLED SUBSTANCE INCLUDED IN SCHEDULE I OF §36-2512 THE MEDICAL DOCTOR SHALL RECEIVE IN WRITING THE CONSENT OF THE PATIENT.

3.ANY FAILURE TO COMPLY WT. THE PROVISIONS OF THIS SECTION MAY BE THE SUBJECT OF INVESTIGATION AND APPROPRIATE DISCIPLINING ACTION BY THE BOARD OF MEDICAL EXAMINERS.

Section 8.

Title 41, Chapter 11, Arizona Revised Statutes, is amended by adding §41-1604.15 to read as follows:

§41-1604.15. PAROLE ELIGIBILITY FOR PERSONS PREVIOUSLY CONVICTED OF PERSONAL POSSESSION OR USE OF A CONTROLLED SUBSTANCE

1.NOTWITHSTANDING ANY LAW TO THE CONTRARY, IF A PRISONER HAS BEEN CONVICTED OF THE PERSONAL POSSESSION OR USE OF A CONTROLLED SUBSTANCE AS DEFINED IN §36-2501, AND IS NOT CONCURRENTLY SERVING ANOTHER SENTENCE, THE PRISONER SHALL BE ELIGIBLE FOR PAROLE.

2.ANY PERSON WHO HAS PREVIOUSLY BEEN CONVICTED OF A VIOLENT CRIME AS DEFINED IN §41-1604.14, SUBSECTION B OR HAS PREVIOUSLY BEEN CONVICTED, SENTENCED OR SUBJECT TO SENTENCING UNDER ANY HABITUAL CRIMINAL STATUTE IN ANY JURISDICTION IN THE UNITED STATES, SHALL NOT BE ELIGIBLE FOR PAROLE PURSUANT TO THE PROVISIONS OF THIS SECTION.

3.PERSONAL POSSESSION OR USE OF A CONTROLLED SUBSTANCE PURSUANT TO THIS ACT SHALL NOT INCLUDE POSSESSION FOR SALE, PRODUCTION, MANUFACTURING, OR TRANSPORTATION FOR SALE OF ANY CONTROLLED SUBSTANCE.

4.WITHIN NINETY (90) DAYS OF THE EFFECTIVE DATE OF THIS ACT, THE DIRECTOR OF THE STATE DEPARTMENT OF CORRECTIONS SHALL PREPARE A LIST WHICH IDENTIFIES EACH PERSON WHO IS ELIGIBLE FOR PAROLE PURSUANT TO THE PROVISIONS OF THIS SECTION, AND DELIVER THE LIST TO THE BOARD OF EXECUTIVE CLEMENCY.

Section 9.

Title 31, Chapter 3, Arizona Revised Statutes, is amended by adding §31-411.01 to read as follows:

§31-411.01. PAROLE FOR PERSONS PREVIOUSLY CONVICTED OF PERSONAL POSSESSION OR USE OF A CONTROLLED SUBSTANCE; TREATMENT; PREVENTION; EDUCATION; TERMINATION OF PAROLE

1.NOTWITHSTANDING ANY LAW TO THE CONTRARY, EVERY PRISONER WHO IS ELIGIBLE FOR PAROLE PURSUANT TO THE PROVISIONS OF §41-1604.15 SHALL BE RELEASED UPON PAROLE, PROVIDED, HOWEVER THAT IF THE BOARD OF EXECUTIVE CLEMENCY DETERMINES THAT A PRISONER SO ELIGIBLE WOULD BE A DANGER TO THE GENERAL PUBLIC, THAT PRISONER SHALL NOT BE RELEASED UPON PAROLE.

2.AS TO EACH PRISONER RELEASED UPON PAROLE PURSUANT TO THE PROVISIONS OF THIS SECTION, THE BOARD SHALL ORDER THAT AS A CONDITION OF PAROLE THE PERSON BE REQUIRED TO PARTICIPATE IN AN APPROPRIATE DRUG TREATMENT OR EDUCATION PROGRAM ADMINISTERED BY A QUALIFIED AGENCY OR ORGANIZATION THAT PROVIDES SUCH TREATMENTS TO PERSONS WHO ABUSE CONTROLLED SUBSTANCES. EACH PERSON ENROLLED IN A DRUG TREATMENT OR EDUCATION PROGRAM SHALL BE REQUIRED TO PAY FOR HIS OR HER PARTICIPATION IN THE PROGRAM TO THE EXTENT OF HIS OR HER FINANCIAL ABILITY.

3.EACH PERSON RELEASED UPON PAROLE PURSUANT TO THE PROVISIONS OF THIS SECTION SHALL REMAIN ON PAROLE UNLESS THE BOARD REVOKES PAROLE OR GRANTS AN ABSOLUTE DISCHARGE FROM PAROLE OR UNTIL THE PRISONER REACHES HIS OR HER INDIVIDUAL EARNED RELEASE CREDIT DATE PURSUANT TO §41-1604.10. WHEN THE PRISONER REACHES HIS OR HER INDIVIDUAL EARNED RELEASE CREDIT DATE, HIS OR HER PAROLE SHALL BE TERMINATED AND HE OR SHE SHALL NO LONGER BE UNDER THE AUTHORITY OF THE BOARD.

Section 10.

Title 13, Chapter 9, Arizona Revised Statutes, is amended by adding §13-901.01 to read as follows:

§13-901.01. PROBATION FOR PERSONS CONVICTED OF PERSONAL POSSESSION AND USE OF CONTROLLED SUBSTANCES; TREATMENT; PREVENTION; EDUCATION

1.NOTWITHSTANDING ANY LAW TO THE CONTRARY, ANY PERSON WHO IS CONVICTED OF THE PERSONAL POSSESSION OR USE OF A CONTROLLED SUBSTANCE AS DEFINED IN §36-2501 SHALL BE ELIGIBLE FOR PROBATION. THE COURT SHALL SUSPEND THE IMPOSITION OR EXECUTION OF SENTENCE AND PLACE SUCH PERSON ON PROBATION.

2.ANY PERSON WHO HAS BEEN CONVICTED OF OR INDICTED FOR A VIOLENT CRIME AS DEFINED §41-1604.14, SUBSECTION B SHALL NOT BE ELIGIBLE FOR PROBATION AS PROVIDED FOR IN THIS SECTION, BUT INSTEAD SHALL BE SENTENCED PURSUANT TO THE OTHER PROVISIONS OF TITLE 13, CHAPTER 34.

3.PERSONAL POSSESSION OR USE OF A CONTROLLED SUBSTANCE PURSUANT TO THIS ACT SHALL NOT INCLUDE POSSESSION FOR SALE, PRODUCTION, MANUFACTURING, OR TRANSPORTATION FOR SALE OF ANY CONTROLLED SUBSTANCE.

4.IF A PERSON IS CONVICTED OF PERSONAL POSSESSION OR USE OF A CONTROLLED SUBSTANCE AS DEFINED IN §36-2501, AS A CONDITION OF PROBATION, THE COURT SHALL REQUIRE PARTICIPATION IN AN APPROPRIATE DRUG TREATMENT OR EDUCATION PROGRAM ADMINISTERED BY A QUALIFIED AGENCY OR ORGANIZATION THAT PROVIDES SUCH PROGRAMS TO PERSONS WHO ABUSE CONTROLLED SUBSTANCES. EACH PERSON ENROLLED IN A DRUG TREATMENT OR EDUCATION PROGRAM SHALL BE REQUIRED TO PAY FOR HIS OR HER PARTICIPATION IN THE PROGRAM TO THE EXTENT OF HIS OR HER FINANCIAL ABILITY.

5.A PERSON WHO HAS BEEN PLACED ON PROBATION UNDER THE PROVISIONS OF THIS SECTION, WHO IS DETERMINED BY THE COURT TO BE IN VIOLATION OF HIS OR HER PROBATION SHALL HAVE NEW CONDITIONS OF PROBATION ESTABLISHED IN THE FOLLOWING MANNER: THE COURT SHALL SELECT THE ADDITIONAL CONDITIONS IT DEEMS NECESSARY, INCLUDING INTENSIFIED DRUG TREATMENT, COMMUNITY SERVICE, INTENSIVE PROBATION, HOME ARREST, OR ANY OTHER SUCH SANCTIONS SHORT OF INCARCERATION.

6.IF PERSON IS CONVICTED A SECOND TIME OF PERSONAL POSSESSION OR USE OF A CONTROLLED SUBSTANCE AS DEFINED IN §36-2501, THE COURT MAY INCLUDE ADDITIONAL CONDITIONS OF PROBATION IT DEEMS NECESSARY, INCLUDING INTENSIFIED DRUG TREATMENT, COMMUNITY SERVICE, INTENSIVE PROBATION, HOME ARREST, OR ANY OTHER ACTION WITHIN THE JURISDICTION OF THE COURT.

7.A PERSON WHO HAS BEEN CONVICTED THREE TIMES OF PERSONAL POSSESSION OR USE OF A CONTROLLED SUBSTANCE AS DEFINED IN §36-2501 SHALL NOT BE ELIGIBLE FOR PROBATION UNDER THE PROVISIONS OF THIS SECTION, BUT INSTEAD SHALL BE SENTENCED PURSUANT TO THE OTHER PROVISIONS OF TITLE 13, CHAPTER 34.

Section 11.

Title 13, Chapter 9, Arizona Revised Statutes, is amended by adding §13-901.02 to read as follows:

§13-901.02. DRUG TREATMENT AND EDUCATION FUND

1.THERE IS HEREBY CREATED A SPECIAL FUND WHICH SHALL BE CALLED THE DRUG TREATMENT AND EDUCATION FUND IN THE ADMINISTRATIVE OFFICE OF SUPREME COURT.

2.FIFTY (50) PERCENT OF THE MONIES DEPOSITED IN THE DRUG TREATMENT AND EDUCATION FUND SHALL BE DISTRIBUTED BY THE ADMINISTRATIVE OFFICE OF THE SUPREME COURT TO THE SUPERIOR COURT PROBATION DEPARTMENTS TO COVER THE COSTS OF PLACING PERSONS IN DRUG EDUCATION AND TREATMENT PROGRAMS ADMINISTERED BY A QUALIFIED AGENCY OR ORGANIZATION THAT PROVIDES SUCH PROGRAMS TO PERSONS WHO ABUSE CONTROLLED SUBSTANCES. SUCH MONIES SHALL BE ALLOCATED TO SUPERIOR COURT PROBATION DEPARTMENTS ACCORDING TO A FORMULA BASED ON PROBATION CASELOAD TO BE ESTABLISHED BY THE ADMINISTRATIVE OFFICE OF THE SUPREME COURT.

3.FIFTY (50) PERCENT OF THE MONIES DEPOSITED IN THE DRUG TREATMENT AND EDUCATION FUND SHALL BE TRANSFERRED TO THE ARIZONA PARENTS COMMISSION ON DRUG EDUCATION AND PREVENTION ESTABLISHED PURSUANT TO §41-1604.16.

4.THE ADMINISTRATIVE OFFICE OF THE SUPREME COURT SHALL CAUSE TO BE PREPARED AT THE END OF EACH FISCAL YEAR AFTER 1997 AN ACCOUNTABILITY REPORT CARD THAT DETAILS THE COST SAVINGS REALIZED FROM THE DIVERSION OF PERSONS FROM PRISONS TO PROBATION. A COPY OF THE REPORT SHALL BE SUBMITTED TO THE GOVERNOR AND THE LEGISLATURE, AND A COPY OF THE REPORT SHALL BE SENT TO EACH PUBLIC LIBRARY IN THE STATE. THE ADMINISTRATIVE OFFICE OF THE SUPREME COURT SHALL RECEIVE REIMBURSEMENT FROM THE DRUG TREATMENT AND EDU-

CATION FUND FOR ANY ADMINISTRATIVE COSTS IT INCURS IN THE IMPLEMENTATION OF THIS ACT.

Section 12.

Title 42, Chapter 12 is amended by adding §42-1204.01 as follows:

§42-1204.01. LUXURY PRIVILEGES TAX; PURPOSE; DRUG TREATMENT AND EDUCATION FUND; DEPARTMENT OF CORRECTIONS REVOLVING FUND

1.NOTWITHSTANDING ANY LAW TO THE CONTRARY, SEVEN (7) PERCENT OF THE MONIES COLLECTED BETWEEN JANUARY 1, 1997 AND DECEMBER 31, 1999, PURSUANT TO §42-1204 SUBSECTION A, PARAGRAPH 1, AND EIGHTEEN (18) PERCENT OF MONIES COLLECTED BETWEEN JANUARY 1, 1997 AND DECEMBER 31, 1999, PURSUANT TO SUBSECTION A, PARAGRAPHS 2, 3, AND 4, SHALL BE DEPOSITED IN THE DRUG TREATMENT AND EDUCATION FUND ESTABLISHED PURSUANT TO §13-902.02.

2.NOTWITHSTANDING ANY LAW TO THE CONTRARY, THREE (3) PERCENT OF THE MONIES COLLECTED BETWEEN JANUARY 1, 1997 AND DECEMBER 31, 1999, PURSUANT TO SECTION §42-1204 SUBSECTION A, PARAGRAPH 1, AND SEVEN (7) PERCENT OF MONIES COLLECTED BETWEEN JANUARY 1, 1997 AND DECEMBER 31, 1999, PURSUANT TO SUBSECTION A, PARAGRAPHS 2, 3. AND 4, SHALL BE DEPOSITED IN A SEPARATE REVOLVING FUND OF THE DEPARTMENT OF CORRECTIONS FOR PAYMENT OF THE EXPENSES OF IMPLEMENTING THE PROVISIONS OF §31-411.01, AND SHALL NOT REVERT TO THE STATE GENERAL FUND IF UNEXPENDED AT THE CLOSE OF THE FISCAL YEAR.

3.NOTWITHSTANDING ANY LAW TO THE CONTRARY, TEN (10) PERCENT OF THE MONIES COLLECTED AFTER DECEMBER 31, 1999 PURSUANT TO §42-1204 SUBSECTION A, PARAGRAPH 1, AND TWENTY FIVE (25) PERCENT OF THE MONIES COLLECTED AFTER DECEMBER 31, 1999 PURSUANT TO SUBSECTION A, PARAGRAPHS 2, 3, AND 4, SHALL BE DEPOSITED IN THE DRUG TREATMENT AND EDUCATION FUND ESTABLISHED PURSUANT TO §13-902.02.

Section 13. Severability

If any provision of this Act, or part thereof, is for any reason held to be invalid or unconstitutional, the remaining sections shall not be affected but shall remain in full force and effect, and to this end the provisions of the Act are severable.

Source of Document: Arizona Office of the Secretary of State

Appendix 3

PROPOSITION 215
MEDICAL MARIJUANA INITIATIVE

Section 1. Section 11362.5 is added to the Health and Safety Code, to read:

11362.5. (a) This section shall be known and may be cited as the Compassionate Use Act of 1996.

(b) (1) The people of the State of California hereby find and declare that the purposes of the Compassionate Use Act of 1996 are as follows:

(A) To ensure that seriously ill Californians have the right to obtain and use marijuana for medical purposes where that medical use is deemed appropriate and has been recommended by a physician who has determined that the person's health would benefit from the use of marijuana in the treatment of cancer, anorexia, AIDS, chronic pain, spasticity, glaucoma, arthritis, migraine, or any other illness for which marijuana provides relief.

(B) To ensure that patients and their primary caregivers who obtain and use marijuana for medical purposes upon the recommendation of a physician are not subject to criminal prosecution or sanction.

(C) To encourage the federal and state governments to implement a plan to provide for the safe and affordable distribution of marijuana to all patients in medical need of marijuana.

(2) Nothing in this act shall be construed to supersede legislation prohibiting persons from engaging in conduct that endangers others, nor to condone the diversion of marijuana for nonmedical purposes.

(c) Notwithstanding any other provision of law, no physician in this state shall be punished, or denied any right or privilege, for having recommended marijuana to a patient for medical purposes.

(d) Section 11357, relating to the possession of marijuana, and Section 11358, relating to the cultivation of marijuana, shall not apply to a patient, or to a patient's primary caregiver, who possesses or cultivates marijuana for the personal medical purposes of the patient upon the written or oral recommendation or approval of a physician.

(e) For the purposes of this section, "primary caregiver" means the individual designated by the person exempted under this act who has consistently assumed responsibility for the housing, health, or safety of that person.

Sec. 2. If any provision of this measure or the application thereof to any person or circumstance is held invalid, that invalidity shall not affect other provisions or applications of the measure which can be given effect without the invalid provision or application, and to this end the provisions of this measure are severable.

Appendix 4

How Can a State Legislature Enable Patients to Use Medicinal Marijuana Despite Federal Prohibition?

Impediments to State Reform Imposed by Federal Law

The Marijuana Tax Act of 1937 established the federal prohibition of marijuana. The American Medical Association testified against the Act, realizing that it would ultimately prevent the medicinal use of marijuana.

The federal Controlled Substances Act of 1970 created a series of five schedules establishing varying degrees of control over certain substances.[1] Marijuana and its primary active ingredient — tetrahydrocannabinol (THC) — are presently in Schedule I, which is defined as follows: "1) The drug or other substance has a high potential for abuse, 2)the drug or other substance has no currently accepted medical use in treatment in the United States, and 3) there is a lack of accepted safety for use of the drug or other substance under medical supervision." As such, doctors may not prescribe marijuana under any circumstances.

The Drug Enforcement Administration (DEA) has been delegated the authority to determine the schedule into which a controlled substance is placed. As a result of years of litigation, it has essentially been determined that the DEA will not move a substance into a less restrictive schedule without an official determination of safety and efficacy by the Food and Drug Administration (FDA). This requires a series of controlled scientific studies.

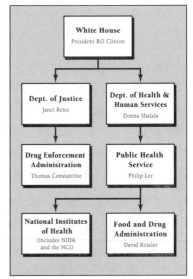

Congress created controlled substance schedules, and Congress has the power to override the DEA and reschedule a substance through legislation. The Attorney General — the executive branch cabinet official who heads the U.S. Department of Justice — also has the authority to override the DEA. However, both of these courses of action are unprecedented.

In 1986, the pill "dronabinol," comprised of synthetic THC in sesame oil in a gelatin capsule, was moved from Schedule I into Schedule II — a slightly less restrictive schedule. Doctors can prescribe dronabinol (marketed as "Marinol") under tightly restricted circumstances, as Schedule II substances are defined as having accepted medical use "with severe restrictions" and having a high potential for abuse and dependence. Schedules III, IV, and V are progressively less restrictive.

The DEA applied special restrictions to dronabinol that do not generally apply to ScheduleII substances: Doctors may be penalized for prescribing dronabinol for conditions other than those "approved" by the FDA — presently, AIDS wasting syndrome and cancer chemotherapy-induced nausea.

While the THC pill provides relief for some patients, others find it inadequate and instead need to use natural marijuana.

Most states mirror the scheduling criteria established by the federal government. However, marijuana has been assigned to Schedule II or lower in a few states that have recognized its medicinal value and/or relative safety. Rescheduling on the state level is mainly symbolic at this time — doctors may not prescribe marijuana in those states because the federal schedules supersede state law.

Regardless of what a state government prefers, marijuana is a Schedule I controlled substance on the federal level. This means that patients are subject to the same penalties as any other marijuana offender. Presently, even for a first offense:

- A patient arrested by federal authorities for possessing even a small amount of marijuana for personal, medicinal use is subject to the same federal penalties as a person who possessed marijuana for recreational use — up to one year in federal prison and a $10,000 fine;[2]

- A patient caught cultivating even one marijuana plant faces up to 5 years in federal prison and a $250,000 fine;[3]
- A patient caught cultivating 100 or more marijuana plants — including seedlings — faces a mandatory minimum of 5 years and a maximum of 40 years in federal prison and a $2 million fine;[4]
- Anyone distributing marijuana to patients — even a registered pharmacist or an official of the state government itself, if outside the auspices of a federally approved research program — can be arrested and tried as a common drug dealer on the federal level. Depending on the amount of marijuana involved, life in prison or even the death penalty may apply![5]

In sum, the federal government prohibits the possession, cultivation, and distribution of marijuana for any reason — including medical use. There is only one exception now available: federally approved research.

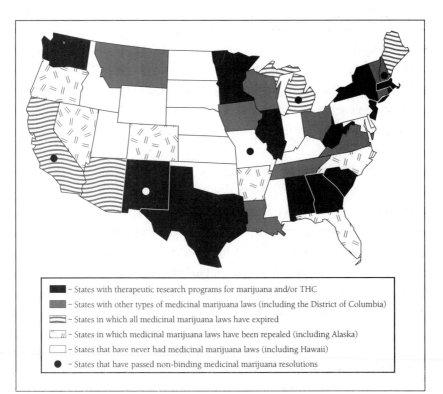

■	– States with therapeutic research programs for marijuana and/or THC
▨	– States with other types of medicinal marijuana laws (including the District of Columbia)
▤	– States in which all medicinal marijuana laws have expired
▨	– States in which medicinal marijuana laws have been repealed (including Alaska)
▢	– States that have never had medicinal marijuana laws (including Hawaii)
●	– States that have passed non-binding medicinal marijuana resolutions

Since the late 1970s, 24 states have passed legislation creating state-run research programs for marijuana and/or THC. (See chart on previous page.) These laws have since expired in six states and been repealed in five states, and they remain on the books in 13 states (and are presently operating in three, California, Arizona and Ohio).

The typical structure of a state program is as follows:

- The program is administered by the state department of health or board of pharmacy;
- Participating patients, physicians, and pharmacies that dispense the marijuana must be approved by a patient qualification review board;
- Patients must be suffering from glaucoma or undergoing cancer chemotherapy or radiology — and not responding or having adverse reactions to conventional treatment;
- In some states, patients with other ailments may participate - but only after receiving special approval from the appropriate agencies;
- The research protocols must be approved by the FDA, and the programs must adhere to federal regulations;
- The marijuana and THC must be supplied by the federal government — but in some states the state department of health or board of pharmacy was permitted to distribute confiscated marijuana to patients in emergency situations;
- Program administrators must collect and analyze data; and
- Patients' privacy must be protected.

Significant variations from this typical structure are explained in the chart.

At least seven states obtained all of the necessary federal permissions, received marijuana and/or THC from NIDA, and distributed the substances to approved patients through approved pharmacies.[6, 7] These states included California, Georgia, Michigan, New Mexico, New York, Tennessee, and Washington.

Though all of these programs have since expired, been repealed, or simply ceased operating, for a brief period of time some of these programs allowed hundreds of patients to use marijuana under their doctors' supervi-

States with CURRENT Medicinal Marijuana Laws

state	schedule (marijuana, THC, dronabinol)	citation for schedules	med. mj law approved	took effect	bill #	session law	citation for med. mj law	description of law
AL	I I	§ 20-2-23(3) and AAC Chap. 420-7-2	July 30, 1979	July 30, 1979	S. 559	Act No 79-472	§ 20-2-110	therapeutic research program

Remarks: For cancer chemotherapy and glaucoma.
State Board of Medical Examiners creates review committee to administer program.
S. 163 (Act. No. 81-506) made minor changes.

state	schedule	citation for schedules	approved	took effect	bill #	session law	citation for med. mj law	description
CT	I I	§ 21a-243 and § 21a-243-7 Reg. of Conn. State Agencies	not available	July 1, 1981	Sub. H.B. 5217	Public Act No. 81-440	§ 21a-246 and § 21a-253	physicians may prescribe

Remarks: For cancer chemotherapy and glaucoma.
Law formerly set out as § 19-453 and § 19-460a, but sections were transferred in 1983; allows physicians licensed by the Commissioner of Consumer Protection to supply marijuana; allows patients to possess marijuana obtained from a prescription, makes no provision for the marijuana supply

| DC | V   II | § 33-516 | June 9, 1981 | August 5, 1981 | Bill No. 4-123 | Law 4-29 (1981) | § 33-522 | scheduling recognizes marijuana's therapeutic use |

Remarks: Marijuana ("cannabis") is listed among the substances in Schedule V, which are found to have a "low potential for abuse," "currently accepted medical use in treatment in the United States or the District of Columbia," and "limited physical dependence or psychological dependence." The 1981 bill, entitled the "District of Columbia Uniform Controlled Substances Act of 1981," replaced a set of controlled substances laws that did not include a scheduling system and did not recognize marijuana's therapeutic uses.

| GA | N/A   II | 16-13-25 | Feb. 22, 1980 | Feb. 22, 1980 | H.B. 1077 | No. 710 (1980) | 43-34-120 and Rules and Regulations Chapter 360-12 | therapeutic research program |

Remarks: For cancer and glaucoma (marijuana or THC).
Composite State Board of Medical Examiners appoints a Patient Qualification Review Board which approves patients, physicians, and pharmacies for participation; no other ailments allowed.

| IA | I*   I* | § 124.204 and § 124.206 | June 1, 1979 | July 1, 1979 | S.F. 487 | Ch. 9 (1979) | § 124.204 and § 124.206 and Administrative Code 620-12 | scheduling recognizes marijuana's therapeutic use |

Remarks: The bill appropriated $247,000 to the Board of Pharmacy Examiners which was contingent upon the Board of Pharmacy Examiners' establishing a therapeutic research program within 90 days of the effective date of the act (July 1, 1979); the board shall organize a Physicians Advisory Group to advise the board on the structure of the program.
*The bill also implemented a dual scheduling scheme for marijuana and THC — marijuana and THC are in Schedule I but are considered to be in Schedule II when used for medicinal purposes.
Scheduling information was originally located at § 204.204 but was moved to § 124.204 in 1993 by the Iowa Code Editor. No disease groups specified in the bill. The dual scheduling scheme still exists in the statutes, but the language for the therapeutic research program existed only in the administrative code from October 1, 1979, to June 30, 1981.

| IL | N/A   II | 720 ILCS 570/206 and 77 IAC Ch. X, Sec. 2070 | September 9, 1978 | September 9, 1978 | H.B. 2625 | 80-1426 | 720 ILCS 550/11 and 77 IAC Ch. X, Sec. 2085 | therapeutic research program |

Remarks: For glaucoma and cancer chemotherapy and radiology or other procedures.
Allows persons "engaged in research" to use marijuana when authorized by physician, must be approved by Department of Mental Health and Developmental Disabilities.

state	schedule (marijuana, THC, dronabinol)			citation for schedules	med. mj law approved	took effect	bill #	session law	citation for med. mj law	description of law
LA	I	I	II	40:964	July 17, 1978; July 23, 1991	August 14, 1978; August 21, 1991	S.B. 245 (1978); H.B. 1187 (1991)	Act No. 725 (1978); Act No. 874 (1991)	40:1021	physicians may prescribe

Remarks: For glaucoma, cancer chemotherapy, and "spastic quadriplegia."
A previous law, 40:1021 - 40:1026, had been repealed by H.B. 1224 in 1989 (Act No. 662). The previous law was a therapeutic research program that addressed only glaucoma and cancer. The present law allows physicians with Schedule I licenses to prescribe marijuana in accordance with regulations promulgated by the Secretary of Health and Hospitals.

state										
MA	N/A	N/A	N/A	94C § 31	Dec. 31, 1991	Dec. 31, 1991	S. 1582	ch. 480 (1991)	94D § 1	therapeutic research program

Remarks: For cancer chemotherapy and radiology, glaucoma, and asthma (marijuana or THC).
Controlled substances are in Classes A, B, C, and D, which determine the severity of penalties for possession, manufacture, and distribution of these substances. The classes make no statement as to the medical value of the controlled substances.
On August 8, 1996, Massachusetts passed a second medicinal marijuana bill (H. 2170) which mandates that within 180 days, the state's public health department must establish the rules and regulations necessary to get its therapeutic research program running and to allow a defense of medical necessity for enrolled patients.

MN	I*		II	§ 152.02 and MR 6800.4200	April 24, 1980	April 25, 1980	H.F. 2476	ch. 614 (1980)	§ 152.21	therapeutic research program

Remarks: For cancer only (research THC only).
The 1980 bill originally appropriated $100,000 to the THC Therapeutic Research Act, but this line-item was vetoed by the governor.
*THC is in Schedule I but is considered to be in Schedule II when used for medicinal purposes.

MT	I		II	50-32-222	March 26, 1979	March 26, 1979	H.B. 463	ch. 320 (1979)	50-32-222(7)	scheduling recognizes marijuana's therapeutic use

Remarks: Would automatically reschedule THC and marijuana to Schedule II if the federal government authorizes the prescription or administration of these substances.

NH	I*	II*		318-B:1-a	April 23, 1981	June 22, 1981	S.B. 21	ch. 107 (1981)	318-B:9	physicians may prescribe

Remarks: For cancer chemotherapy and radiology.
*State follows the federal government's scheduling of controlled substances as articulated in the Code of Federal Regulations [318-B:1-a; June 11, 1996, phone conversation with John McCormick at New Hampshire State Library, 603-271-2239].

NJ	I		II	24:21-5 and 8:65-10 New Jersey Administrative Code	March 23, 1981	March 23, 1981	A.B. 819	ch. 72 (1981)	26:2L	therapeutic research program

Remarks: For life- or sense-threatening diseases.
Pertains to any Schedule I substance (not specific to marijuana); administered by Department of Health; only for patients participating in research programs conducted by FDA; patients and physicians certified by Therapeutic Research Qualification Board; get substances from NIDA.

NM	I*	II*		30-31-3	Feb. 21, 1978	Feb. 21, 1978	H.B. 329	ch. 22 (1978)	26-2A	therapeutic research program

Remarks: For glaucoma and cancer chemotherapy (marijuana or THC); patients with other diseases must get approval from Patient Qualification Review Board.
Administered by the Department of Health and Environment; marijuana and THC considered to be in Schedule II when dispensed through the program.
Would have expired on July 1, 1979, but ch. 11 (1979) extended the program indefinitely.
*State follows the federal government's scheduling of controlled substances as articulated in the Code of Federal Regulations [30-31-5; Board of Pharmacy, 505-841-9102]. Marijuana and THC are in Schedule I but are considered to be in Schedule II when used for medicinal purposes.

state	schedule (marijuana, THC, dronabinol)	citation for schedules	med. mj law approved	took effect	bill #	session law	citation for med. mj law	description of law
NY	I II	PHL § 3306	June 30, 1980	Sept. 1, 1980	S.B. 1123-6	ch. 810 (1980)	PHL § 3397 and PHL § 3328	therapeutic research program

Remarks: For cancer, glaucoma, and other life- and sense-threatening diseases approved by the commissioner. Administered by Department of Health and Patient Qualification Review Board; confiscated marijuana may be used if necessary.

In 1981, the name of the "controlled substances therapeutic research program" was changed to the "Antonio G. Olivieri controlled substances therapeutic research program" by ch. 208 (1981).

| OH | I   II | § 3719.41 | March 21, 1980; not available | June 20, 1980; July 1, 1996 | S.B. 184; S.B. 2 | Act No. 230 (1980); not available | § 2925.11(I) | medical necessity defense |

Remarks: 1980 law which expired on June 20, 1984, was a therapeutic research program administered by Director of Health; marijuana and THC; Patient Review Board; glaucoma, cancer chemotherapy or radiology, or other medical conditions; law appeared at § 3719.85.

The 1996 law reads as follows: "It is an affirmative defense ... to a charge of possessing marijuana under this section that the offender, pursuant to the prior written recommendation of a licensed physician, possessed the marijuana solely for medicinal purposes."

| RI | I   II | § 21-28-2.08 | May 19, 1980 | May 19, 1980 | H.B. 79.6072 | ch. 375 (1980) | § 21-28.4-1 | therapeutic research program |

Remarks: Patients must be involved in a life- or sense-threatening situation (original law specified cancer chemotherapy, glaucoma, and other disease groups); program administered by director of the Department of Health; director or director's designee reviews patients and physicians for participation in program (original law specified Patient Qualification Review Board). Amended by 86-H 7817 in 1986 (ch. 236) to instead say "life- or sense-threatening conditions," and deletes references to Patient Qualification Review Board.

| SC | I   II* | § 44-53-160 and § 44-53-190 | Feb. 28, 1980 | Feb. 28, 1980 | S. 350 | Act No. 323 (1980) | § 44-53-610 | therapeutic research program |

Remarks: For glaucoma and cancer chemotherapy and radiology and other disease groups (marijuana and THC). Administered by commissioner of Department of Health and Environmental Control and patient qualification review advisory board; "Commissioner shall obtain marijuana through whatever means he deems most appropriate consistent with federal law."

Minor amendments made by Act No. 181 (1993).

*State follows the federal government's scheduling of controlled substances as articulated in the Code of Federal Regulations [§ 44-53-160].

| TN | I   VI*   II | § 39-17-408 | April 2, 1981 | April 2, 1981 | H.B. 314 | ch. 114 (1981) | § 68-52-101 | scheduling recognizes marijuana's therapeutic use |

Remarks: The bill created a therapeutic research program for cancer chemotherapy or radiology or glaucoma (marijuana or THC); administered by Patient Qualification Review Board created within Board of Pharmacy; PQRB shall contract with federal government for marijuana.

Therapeutic research program repealed by S.B. 1818 in 1992 (ch. 537), but dual scheduling scheme still remains.

*Marijuana and THC are in Schedule VI but are considered to be in Schedule II when used for medicinal purposes. (Schedule VI includes controlled substances that "should not be included in Schedules I through V." Schedules I through V have the typical definitions used in other states.)

state	schedule (marijuana, THC, dronabinol)			citation for schedules	med. mj law approved	took effect	bill #	session law	citation for med. mj law	description of law
TX	I	I*		H & S § 481.032 and § 481.038 and 37 TAC § 13.1	June 14, 1979	January 1, 1980	S.B. 877	ch. 826 (1979)	H & S §§ 481.111 and § 481.201-205	therapeutic research program

Remarks: For cancer and glaucoma (THC or its derivatives).
Administered by Board of Health and Research Program Review Board; RPRB, after approval of Board of Health, may seek authorization to expand research program to include other diseases; get THC from federal government.
Minor amendments made by S.B. 688 in 1983 (ch. 566). H.B. 2136 in 1989 (ch. 678) moved the therapeutic research program law from Civil Statutes Health Art. 4476-15 to H & S §§ 481.201-205.
*State follows the federal government's scheduling of controlled substances as articulated in the Code of Federal Regulations [H & S § 481.038].

state	schedule (marijuana, THC, dronabinol)			citation for schedules	med. mj law approved	took effect	bill #	session law	citation for med. mj law	description of law
VA	N/A	I	II	§ 54.1-3443	March 27, 1979	Spring 1979	S. 913	ch. 435 (1979)	§§ 18.2-250.1 and § 18.2-251.1	physicians may prescribe

Remarks: For cancer and glaucoma (marijuana or THC).
Allows physicians to prescribe and pharmacists to dispense marijuana and THC for such purposes.

state	schedule (marijuana, THC, dronabinol)			citation for schedules	med. mj law approved	took effect	bill #	session law	citation for med. mj law	description of law
VT	N/A	N/A	N/A	N/A	April 27, 1981	April 27, 1981	H. 130	Act No. 49 (1981)	18 VSA § 4471	physicians may prescribe

Remarks: For cancer and other medicinal uses as determined by the Commissioner of Health.
Administered by Department of Health; called a "research program" but really enables physicians to prescribe marijuana; "commissioner of health shall have the authority to obtain ... cannabis administered under this program."

state	schedule (marijuana, THC, dronabinol)			citation for schedules	med. mj law approved	took effect	bill #	session law	citation for med. mj law	description of law
WA	I	II		69.50.204 and WAC 246-887-100	March 27, 1979	March 27, 1979	H.B. 259	ch. 136 (1979)	69.51	therapeutic research program

Remarks: For cancer chemotherapy and radiology and glaucoma, and other disease groups.
Dual scheduling for marijuana and every compound (including THC) in the marijuana plant; administered by Board of Pharmacy and Patient Qualification Review Committee; "Board shall obtain marijuana through whatever means it deems most appropriate and consistent with regulations promulgated by federal government"; "board may use marijuana which has been confiscated by local or state law enforcement agencies and has been determined to be free from contamination."
Amendment in 1986 (ch. 124) removed the dual scheduling of marijuana and THC; minor amendments made in 1989 (ch. 9).
On March 30, 1996, Washington State enacted the 1996 supplemental operating budget which allocated $130,000 for two medicinal marijuana-related projects: $70,000 to research a tamper-free means of cultivating marijuana for medicinal purposes, and $60,000 to research the therapeutic potential of marijuana.

state	schedule (marijuana, THC, dronabinol)			citation for schedules	med. mj law approved	took effect	bill #	session law	citation for med. mj law	description of law
WI	I	II		161.13; 161.41(3r)	not available; April 20, 1988	April 20, 1982; April 28, 1988	A.B. 697; A.B. 662	ch. 193 (1981); Act 339 (1987)	46.60	physicians may prescribe

Remarks: No disease groups specified (marijuana or THC).
Allows medicinal marijuana prescriptions in accordance with federal IND permits; gives controlled substances board the authority to set up regulations.
A.B. 662 in 1987 (Act 339), enacted in 1988, allows for the possession of THC if obtained directly from a valid prescription.

state	schedule (marijuana, THC, dronabinol)			citation for schedules	med. mj law approved	took effect	bill #	session law	citation for med. mj law	description of law
WV	I	II		§ 60A-2-204	March 10, 1979	June 8, 1979	S.B. 366	ch. 56 (1979)	§ 16-5A-7	therapeutic research program

Remarks: For cancer chemotherapy and glaucoma.
Program administered by director of the Department of Health and Patient Qualification Review Board. PQRB certifies the participation of patients, physicians, and pharmacies for participation in the program; may include other disease groups if approved; director shall contract with federal government for supply of marijuana.

States in which Medicinal Marijuana Laws Have EXPIRED

state	schedule (marijuana, THC, dronabinol)			citation for schedules	med. mj law approved	took effect	bill #	session law	citation for med. mj law	description of law	law expired
AZ	I	II	N/A	§ 36-2512	April 22, 1980	April 22, 1980	H.B. 2020	Ch. 122 (1980)	§ 36-2601	therapeutic research program	expired June 30, 1985
Remarks:	For cancer and glaucoma (marijuana or THC). Director of the Department of Health Services appoints a Patient Qualification Review Board; PQRB reviews patients and doctors for participation in the program; University of Arizona shall obtain marijuana or THC from NIDA. S.B. 1023 in 1981 (ch. 264) moved the therapeutic research program provisions from § 36-1031 to § 36-2601. Had a dual scheduling scheme for marijuana only, but the provisional Schedule II marijuana provision was ultimately replaced with a permanent Schedule II provision for THC. Presumably, dronabinol is considered to be in Schedule II because THC — dronabinol's only active ingredient — is in Schedule II.										
CA	I	II		H & S § 11054	July 25, 1979	July 25, 1979	S.B. 184	Ch. 300 (1979)	H & S § 11260 and H & S § 11480	therapeutic research program	H & S § 11260 would have expired on June 30, 1985, but program was extended and modified slightly by ch. 417 (1984); program finally expired on June 30, 1989; § 11480 is still on the books
Remarks:	For cancer and glaucoma. Research Advisory Panel coordinates research with marijuana and its derivatives; may utilize marijuana from other sources, including seized and forfeited marijuana, if supply is not available from federal government; appropriates $100,000 for first year. Minor amendments by ch. 374 (1980) and ch. 101 (1983).										
ME	N/A	N/A	N/A	17-A § 1102	Sept. 14, 1979; Sept. 23, 1983	Sept. 14, 1979; Sept. 23, 1983	H.B. 665 (1979); H.B. 1025 (1983)	ch. 457 (1979); ch. 423 (1983)	22 § 2401-2410; 22 § 2411-2420	therapeutic research program	1979 law expired in 1981; 1983 law expired in 1987
Remarks:	For glaucoma and cancer chemotherapy. Research program within Department of Human Services; use federal marijuana or, if necessary, marijuana confiscated by state law-enforcement agencies; Participation Review Board approves physicians. Controlled substances are in Schedules W, X, Y, and Z, which determine the severity of penalties for possession, manufacture, and distribution of these substances. The schedules make no statement as to the medical value of the controlled substances.										
MI	I	II		§ 333.7212; MAC 338.3114 and 338.3119a (1986 Annual Supplement); MAC 338.3113 (1988 Annual Supplement)	Oct. 22, 1979; Dec. 21, 1982	Oct. 22, 1979; Dec. 21, 1982	S.B. 185 (1979); S.B. 816 (1982)	Act No. 125 (1979); Act No. 352 (1982)	§ 333.7335	therapeutic research program	1979 law expired November 1, 1982; 1982 law does not apply after November 1, 1987
Remarks:	For glaucoma and cancer chemotherapy (marijuana or THC); allows patients with other diseases if patients have IND permit from FDA. Administered by the Department of Public Health; marijuana and THC considered to be in Schedule II when dispensed through the program; use federal marijuana or, if necessary, marijuana confiscated by state law-enforcement agencies. 1979 law expired on November 1, 1982, and then a nearly identical law was enacted a month later, which expired on November 1, 1987.										

States in which Medicinal Marijuana Laws Have Been REPEALED

state	schedule marijuana	schedule THC	schedule dronabinol	citation for schedules	med. mj law approved	took effect	bill #	session law	citation for med. mj law	description of law	law repealed
AK	VIA	IIIA	IIIA	§ 11.71.160	Spring 1982	Jan. 1, 1983	info not available	§ 5 ch. 45 (1982)	§ 17.35	therapeutic research program	repealed by ch. 146 (1986)
AR	VI	VI	II	§ 5-64-215	Jan. 30, 1981	Jan. 30, 1981	H.B. 171	Act No. 8 (1981)	§ 82-1007 (numbering system has changed since law was repealed)	physicians may prescribe	repealed by Act No. 52 (1987) which also moved dronabinol to Schedule II
CO	N/A	I	II	§ 18-18-203	June 21, 1979	June 21, 1979	H.B. 1042	ch. 265 (1979)	§ 25-5-901 to -907	therapeutic research program	repealed by H.B. 95-1020 in 1995 (ch. 71)
FL	I	I	II	§ 893.03	June 26, 1978	July 1, 1978	H.B. 1237	c. 78-413 (1978)	§ 402.36	therapeutic research program	repealed by c. 84-115 (1984)
NC	VI	VI	II	§ 90-90	June 5, 1979	June 5, 1979	H.B. 1065	ch. 781 (1979)	§ 90-101	physicians may prescribe	de facto repealed by H.B. 878 in 1987 (ch. 412), which allows physicians to administer only dronabinol for cancer chemotherapy

Remarks: For cancer chemotherapy and radiology; and glaucoma. Administered by Board of Pharmacy; patients certified by Patient Qualification Review Committee; Board of Pharmacy may include other disease groups if physician presents pertinent medical data. Marijuana, which is a Schedule VIA drug, has the "lowest degree of danger or probable danger to a person or the public."

Remarks: For cancer (lawfully obtained THC). Marijuana and THC are listed in Schedule VI, but Schedule VI substances are defined similarly — yet even more restrictively — than Schedule I substances.

Remarks: For cancer and glaucoma. Pharmacy and Therapeutics Committee at University of Colorado administers program; PTC may include other disease groups after pertinent data have been presented by physician; apply to receive marijuana from NIDA; if unable to obtain marijuana from NIDA, investigate feasibility of using seized marijuana that has been tested for impurities; appropriates $15,000. Amended by ch. 322 (1981) to say that other disease groups can be included after pertinent data are presented by physician who has an IND number issued by FDA; apply to receive marijuana from federal government.

Remarks: For cancer and glaucoma (marijuana or THC). Program administered by Secretary of Department of Health and Rehabilitative Services who delegates to Patient Qualification Review Board which approves cancer and glaucoma patients; PQRB may include other disease groups after pertinent data have been presented by physician; Secretary of HRS shall apply to federal government for marijuana and shall transfer marijuana to certified state-operated pharmacies for distribution to certified patients upon written prescription of certified physicians. Minor modifications: c. 79-209 (1979), c. 81-279 (1981); interesting modification with c. 82-12 (1982), which changed name from "controlled substances therapeutic research" to "cancer therapeutic research" to allow for "unconventional therapies" that are not yet approved by the federal government.

Remarks: "A physician ... may possess, dispense or administer tetrahydrocannabinols in duly constituted pharmaceutical form for human administration for treatment purposes pursuant to rules adopted by the [North Carolina Drug] Commission." Schedule VI (§ 90-94) is specific to marijuana: "no currently accepted medical use in the United States, or a relatively low potential for abuse in terms of risk to public health and potential to produce psychic or physiological dependence liability based upon present medical knowledge, or a need for further and continuing study to develop scientific evidence of its pharmacological effects."

state	schedule (marijuana, THC, dronabinol)			citation for schedules	med. mj law approved	took effect	bill #	session law	citation for med. mj law	description of law	law repealed
NV	I	I	II	453.510 NAC	June 2, 1979	June 2, 1979	S.B. 470	ch. 610 (1979)	453.740 - 453.810 and 453.740 NAC	therapeutic research program	repealed by A.B. 695 in 1987 (ch. 417)

Remarks: For glaucoma or cancer chemotherapy or others (marijuana and THC).
Administered by Health Division of Department of Human Services; Board of Review for Patients.

state											
OR	I	I	II	475.035 and OAR 855-80	June 18, 1979	June 18, 1979	H.B. 2267	ch. 253 (1979)	475.505 - 475.515	physicians may prescribe	repealed by S.B. 160 in 1987 (ch. 75)

Remarks: For cancer chemotherapy and glaucoma (seized marijuana).
Oregon State Police shall make confiscated marijuana available to the Health Division to test it for contaminants; if marijuana is found to be free of contaminants, Health Division shall make marijuana available to physicians upon written request; patients who are prescribed such marijuana may possess less than an ounce.

States That Have NEVER HAD Medicinal Marijuana Laws

state	schedule (marijuana, THC, dronabinol)			citation for schedules
DE	I		II	16 § 4713
HI	I		II	§ 329-14
ID	I		II	37-2705
IN	I		II	35-48-2
KS	I		II	65-4105
KY	I		II	218A and 902 KAR 55-020
MD	I		II*	27 § 279

* State follows the federal government's scheduling of controlled substances as articulated in the Code of Federal Regulations [27 § 278(c); Dept. of Health and Mental Hygiene, Division of Drug Control, 410-764-2890].

state				
MO	I		II	195.017
MS	I		II	§ 41-29-113
ND	I		II	19-03.1-04
NE	I		II	§ 28-405
OK	I		N/A*	63 § 2-204

* Presumably, dronabinol is considered to be in Schedule II because THC — dronabinol's only active ingredient — is in Schedule II.

state				
PA	I		II	35 § 780-104 and 28 § 25.72 Penn. Code
SD	N/A		II	§ 34-20B-11
UT	I		I	58-37-4
WY	I		II	§ 35-7-1012 and 024 059 101 Wyoming Rules

States That Have Passed Non-Binding Resolutions Urging the Federal Government to Make Marijuana Medically Available

state	res. passed	resolution #
CA	Sept. 2, 1993	Sen. Joint Res. No. 8
MI	March 17, 1982	Sen. Conc. Res. No. 473
MO	Spring 1994	Sen. Conc. Res 14
NH	not available	not available
NM	not available	not available

NOTES:

1. Some states use the spelling "marihuana" in their statutes — "marijuana" is used in this report.
2. Italics for a citation indicates that it is in the state's administrative code (developed by state agencies in the executive branch), not the state's statutes (laws passed by the state legislature).
3. The definitions of Schedule I and Schedule II in state controlled substances acts are always similar to the federal definitions, which can be found on the first page of this report. When marijuana, THC, or dronabinol are not in Schedule I or Schedule II, a clarifying description is noted.
4. THC is an abbreviation for tetrahydrocannabinol, the only active ingredient in marijuana.
5. Dronabinol is an FDA-approved prescription drug (trade name is Marinol) which is defined as THC "in sesame oil and encapsulated in a soft gelatin capsule in a U.S. Food and Drug Administration approved drug product." 21 CFR Sec. 1308.12(f)(1).
6. Trivial amendments are not listed; bills that make minor, non-trivial amendments are listed.
7. Three columns of schedules: "N/A" simply means substance is not scheduled in state statutes or administrative code.
8. Statute citations for medicinal marijuana laws. The administrative code provisions for the therapeutic research programs are cited when possible but are not necessarily cited for all such states. The statute and administrative code citations are for the most recent statute supplements available in the Library of Congress' law library reading room as of June 1996. In some states, the most recent statute supplements were from 1994, and the administrative code citations are generally even more outdated than the statutes.
9. Many states have used a dual scheduling scheme for marijuana and/or THC. In these states, marijuana and THC are in Schedule I but are considered to be in Schedule II when used for medicinal purposes.

sion. The end of these programs' operations coincided with the federal approval of dronabinol, the THC pill, as a prescription medicine.

Typically, patients were referred to the program by their personal physicians. These patients, who had not been responding well to conventional treatments, underwent medical and psychological screening processes. Then the patients applied to the state's patient qualification review board. If granted permission, they would receive marijuana from approved pharmacies. Patients were required to monitor their usage and its effects, which the state used to prepare reports for the FDA.

These programs were designed to enable patients to use marijuana. The research was not intended to generate data that would lead to FDA approval of marijuana as a prescription medicine. For example, the protocols did not involve double-blind assignment to research and control groups. Only one state program — in New York — led to a published journal article.[8]

It is possible that such programs operated in more than seven of the 24 states that passed legislation establishing research programs. This information is not available through the usual research channels, so the MPP filed a Freedom of Information Act request with the FDA and the National Cancer Institute (NCI) on July 15, 1996. Activists who need more detailed information before the MPP receives the documentation from the FDA and/or NCI should contact their state health departments.

The advantages of state therapeutic research programs include:

- Patients in a well-run program have legal access to an inexpensive, unadulterated supply of marijuana;
- Data can be generated that may eventually lead to FDA approval of marijuana as a prescription medicine;
- Laws providing for these programs are still on the books in 13 states. A legislative allocation of money and/or a directive to a state's department of public health may be all it would take to get a program up and running in these states; and
- The programs send a strong message that states want patients to have access to marijuana.

The disadvantages of such programs include:

- It can be a challenge for a state to secure all of the necessary federal permissions. Indeed, most states that passed the necessary laws never implemented the programs;
- Federal bureaucracies were not very cooperative even with the legally operating programs — for example, promised supplies sometimes never arrived;
- It is a bureaucratic hassle for patients to participate in the program;
- There is a very short list of ailments that may qualify a patient for participation — usually cancer and glaucoma;
- The programs may cost each state more than $100,000 annually to pay government employees at the state board of pharmacy to obtain FDA and DEA approval; apply to NIDA for marijuana; approve participating patients, doctors and pharmacies; and otherwise oversee the program;
- The existence of a program — or even a law providing for its creation — may lead a state's courts to rule against allowing the defense of medical necessity. (See next subsection.)

Several state legislatures are again taking an interest in therapeutic research programs, almost always as a direct result of concerted state-level activism.

On March 30, 1996, Washington State Governor Mike Lowry signed into law a state budget allocating $130,000 to two medicinal marijuana-related projects:

- $70,000 will be spent on researching a tamper-free means of cultivating marijuana plants to be used for medicinal purposes. This could result in an application to the federal government to become an alternative source of marijuana for research purposes.
- $60,000 will be spent on researching the effects of medicinal marijuana. This could result in the re-opening of the state's therapeutic research program.

Persuading a state government to start growing its own marijuana would break NIDA's monopoly on the supply and open the doors for more widespread scientific research, bringing FDA-approved prescriptive access one step closer. Of course, the state government must first obtain federal permission to grow marijuana.

A Massachusetts law enacted on August 8, 1996, contains a provision mandating that within 180 days, the state's public health department must establish the rules and regulations necessary to get its therapeutic research program running. This program was provided for in a 1991 law, but no action had been taken to get it running.

Additionally, in 1992 the Maine legislature passed a bill (H.P. 1729/L.D. 2420) which intended to implement a therapeutic research program — it authorized physicians to "prescribe" marijuana in accordance with federal regulations, so it probably would not have been workable — but Governor John McKernan vetoed the bill.

MEDICAL NECESSITY DEFENSE. The earliest method through which state governments — specifically the courts, not legislatures — recognized the medicinal use of marijuana and protected some patients from punishment was through allowing arrested patients to use the affirmative defense of "medical necessity."

The necessity defense, long recognized in common law, gives a defendant the chance to prove in court that his or her violation of the law was necessary to avert a greater evil. This defense may lead to an acquittal, even if the evidence proves that the patient did indeed possess or cultivate marijuana.

Some states have statutes that authorize the "necessity defense" and have specified elements of proof needed to succeed. But this does not guarantee that the courts will recognize a medical necessity defense for marijuana.

If the defense is not recognized, the case proceeds as if the defendant possessed marijuana for recreational purposes or distribution. If found guilty, the offender is subject to prison time in most states.

The medical necessity defense is a very limited, damage-control measure. Though a legislature may codify the defense into law, this is typically not the best course of action for a state legislature to pursue.

The first successful use of the medical necessity defense in a marijuana cultivation case led to the 1976 acquittal of a glaucoma patient in Washington, D.C.[9]

In this case, the court determined that the defense would not have been available if: (1) the defendant had caused the compelling circumstances leading to the violation of the law; (2) a less offensive alternative were available; or (3) the harm avoided were less serious than the conduct to avoid it, i.e., cultivating marijuana.

Courts in at least three other states subsequently allowed the medical necessity defense in medicinal marijuana cases: Washington,[10] Florida,[11] and Idaho.[12]

Unfortunately, other state courts have refused to allow this defense:

- In 1986, the New Jersey Supreme Court ruled that the state legislature — by placing marijuana into Schedule I — had already indicated its legislative intent to prohibit the medicinal use of marijuana. In addition, the court claimed that the criteria of "necessity" could not be met because there were research program options that could have been pursued instead.[13]

- In 1978, the Georgia Court of Appeals ruled that the lack of any medicinal marijuana recognition by the state legislature precluded the court from allowing the medical necessity defense.[14]

- In 1991, the Massachusetts Supreme Judicial Court ruled that the societal harm of allowing the medical necessity defense would be greater than the harm done to a patient denied the opportunity to offer the defense.[15]

- In 1991, the Minnesota Court of Appeals refused to allow a patient to use the medical necessity defense because the legislature had already expressed its intent by placing marijuana in Schedule I — and by establishing a therapeutic research program, thereby directly establishing the very limited circumstances under which marijuana may be used.[16]

- Most recently, in 1993, the Alabama Court of Criminal Appeals used the same reasoning as the Minnesota court to refuse to allow the defense.[17]

These cases demonstrate that, although it is up to the courts to decide whether to allow the medical necessity defense, the activities of a state legislature may significantly impact this decision. Therefore, codifying the medical necessity defense into state law is a valid option for state-level medicinal marijuana activists to consider.

The main advantages of a state's recognition of the medical necessity defense are:

- Some patients may establish their own supply of marijuana — buying it through the criminal market or cultivating their own — without needing to get involved with any bureaucratic regimens; and
- Patients who live in states with no research programs, who have not heard about such programs, or who do not meet the criteria for enrollment in such programs may still avoid prison sentences for using their medicine, even if caught.

The disadvantages of relying exclusively on a state's recognition of the medical necessity defense are:

- It is very difficult to meet the criteria necessary to utilize the defense, so patients with legitimate medical need may still lose their cases;
- Careful documentation of a patient's medical progress and an ongoing collaboration with his or her doctor is necessary to start building a case before the patient is arrested. This can be even more grueling than participating in a research program;
- It doesn't prevent patients from being arrested and put on trial;
- The supply of marijuana is neither truly legal, nor necessarily safe or affordable.

The MPP has identified only three states in which the legislature has passed legislation to establish the medical necessity defense for medicinal marijuana offenses — Maine, Massachusetts, and Ohio.

In 1992, the Maine legislature passed a bill (H.P.1729/L.D. 2420) that, among other things, would have allowed the medical necessity defense for cultivation. As stated previously in this paper, Governor John McKernan vetoed this bill.

In 1994, a bill (H. 3911) introduced in the Massachusetts House of Representatives would have established a "medical necessity defense" as legitimate grounds for acquittal on marijuana possession charges. The bill did not pass the legislature.

Another medical necessity defense bill (H.2170) passed the Massachusetts legislature in 1995 but Governor Bill Weld "returned" it to the legislature, arguing that it was too broad and likely to be abused. A revised version of the bill was signed into law by Gov. Weld on August 8, 1996. The bill, H. 2170, was carefully tailored by the legislature to address his concerns — making it much more limited. The new Massachusetts law expands upon its 1991 therapeutic research program. (See chart and previous subsection.)

The new law would allow patients to use the necessity defense, but only if they are "certified to participate" in the therapeutic research program and possessed the marijuana "for personal use pursuant to such program."

This hardly establishes a meaningful necessity defense: First, it is unimaginable that a patient receiving marijuana as part of this program would ever be arrested for marijuana possession — much less prosecuted and convicted — even without a codified medical necessity defense. Second, the state public health department has failed to launch a program during the five years since the research program law took effect! Presently, there is no such program running in Massachusetts.

Hopefully, the new law will be beneficial anyway because it does raise the possibility that courts may accept a defense of medical necessity for a broader pool of patients — for example, patients who meet the criteria for the program but are not yet enrolled because the program has not started running or because they did not know about it.

In 1995, Ohio Governor George Voinovich signed a comprehensive criminal justice reform bill (S.B. 2) — effective July 1, 1996 — which establishes that "It is an affirmative defense . . . to a charge of possessing marihuana . . . that the offender, pursuant to the prior written recommendation of a licensed physician, possessed the marihuana solely for medicinal purposes." This is the first medicinal marijuana law enacted in Ohio since the state's therapeutic research program expired in 1984. Ohio is the only state to have enacted an effective medical necessity law for marijuana.

Additionally, a 1995 Minnesota bill (H.F. 1136) would have, among other things, provided for a medical necessity defense for marijuana possession. While the bill enjoyed bipartisan support, it was not deemed to be a high enough priority to act upon and died when the legislature adjourned in mid-1996.

Finally, a 1995 Kansas Bill (S.B. 333) included the following provision when it passed the House but which was subsequently removed before the bill passed the full legislature: "It shall be a defense to a prosecution . . . that the person in possession or control of marijuana or tetrahydrocannabinol . . . has been certified to be undergoing treatment for multiple sclerosis or glaucoma or to be undergoing radiation or chemotherapy treatment for cancer by two persons who are licensed to practice medicine and surgery."

There simply are not enough federal (DEA) agents to hunt down and arrest many patients for growing a few marijuana plants. During Alcohol Prohibition, New York and other states repealed the state laws criminalizing alcohol, putting the enforcement burden entirely on the federal government. This eventually led to the repeal of Alcohol Prohibition on the federal level.

To date, no state has removed its penalties for possessing and/or cultivating marijuana for therapeutic use. The likely advantages of such a law would be:

• Patients — and perhaps their caregivers — would be able to supply their own marijuana without fear of arrest or prosecution;

• Unlike the medical necessity defense, patients would merely need to verify to the police or prosecutor that there is a legitimate medical need for marijuana and no further legal proceedings would be necessary. A simple note from a doctor could suffice. On the state level, medicinal marijuana use would be "legal" for individual patients;

- Unlike the therapeutic research programs, no federal bureaucratic red tape would be necessary (and a wider variety of ailments may qualify); and

- A tremendously powerful message would be sent to the federal government, blatantly rejecting its war on patients.

The likely disadvantages would be:

- Federal authorities could still arrest patients, and overzealous state and local police might consider arresting patients and turning them over to federal authorities;

- There would be little or no quality control over the supply of marijuana, since patients would be producing it themselves or getting it from the criminal market;

- Sufficient data for FDA approval of medicinal marijuana would not be generated; and

- Some state governments might be reluctant to pass such sweeping reforms.

All in all, however, the removal of penalties would be the ideal legislation for a state to enact.

. . . .

1. The criteria for each of the schedules, listed in Title 21 of the U.S. Code, Section 812(b) (21 U.S.C. 812(b)), and a few example substances from Title21 of the Code of Federal Regulations, Section 1308, are:

   Schedule I (includes heroin, LSD, and marijuana)

   A. The drug or other substance has a high potential for abuse.

   B. The drug or other substance has no currently accepted medical use in treatment in the United States.

   C. There is a lack of accepted safety for use of the drug or other substance under medical supervision.

   Schedule II (includes morphine, used as a pain-killer, and cocaine, used as a topical anesthetic)

   A. The drug or other substance has a high potential for abuse.

   B. The drug or other substance has a currently accepted medical use in treatment in the United States or a currently accepted medical use with severe restrictions.

   C. Abuse of the drug or other substance may lead to severe psychological or physical dependence.

   Schedule III (includes anabolic steroids)

   A. The drug or other substance has a potential for abuse less than the drugs or other substances in Schedules I and II.

B. The drug or other substance has a currently accepted medical use in treatment in the United States.

C. Abuse of the drug or other substance may lead to moderate or low physical dependence or high psychological dependence.

Schedule IV (includes Valium and other tranquilizers)

A. The drug or other substance has a low potential for abuse relative to the drugs or other substances in Schedule III.

B. The drug or other substance has a currently accepted medical use in treatment in the United States.

C. Abuse of the drug or other substance may lead to limited physical dependence or psychological dependence relative to the drugs or other substances in Schedule III.

Schedule V (includes codeine-containing analgesics)

A. The drug or other substance has a low potential for abuse relative to the drugs or other substances in Schedule IV.

B. The drug or other substance has a currently accepted medical use in treatment in the United States.

C. Abuse of the drug or other substance may lead to limited physical dependence or psychological dependence relative to the drugs or other substances in Schedule IV.

2. 21 U.S.C. 844.

3. 21 U.S.C. 841(b)(1)(D).

4. 21 U.S.C. 841(b)(1)(B).

5. 18 U.S.C. 3591(b).

6. Marijuana, Medicine & the Law, Volume II, R. C. Randall, ed.; Washington, D.C.: Galen Press, 1989.

7. "The Controlled Substances Therapeutic Research Act in the State of Washington," Journal of Clinical Pharmacology, 21; R.A. Roffman, 1981.

8. "Inhalation Marijuana as an Antiemetic of Cancer Chemotherapy," New York State Journal of Medicine; V. Vinciguerra,M.D., October 1988.

9. United States v. Randall, 104 Wash. Daily L. Rep. 2249 (D.C. Super. Ct. 1976).

10. Washington v. Diana, 604 P.2d 1312 (Ct. App. Wash. 1979); Washington v. Cole, 874 P. 2d 878 (Ct. App. Wash. 1994).

11. Florida v. Musikka, No. 88-4395 CFA (17th Judicial Cir. Broward County, Dec. 28, 1988); Jenks v. Florida, 582 So. 2d 676 (Ct. App. 1st Dist., Fl. 1991).

12. Idaho v. Hastings, 801 P. 2d 563 (Sup. Ct. Idaho 1990).

13. New Jersey v. Tate, 505 A. 2d 941 (1986).

14. Spillers v. Georgia, 245 S.E. 2d 54, 55 (1978).

15. Massachusetts v. Hutchins, 575 N.E. 2d 741, 742 (1991).

16. Minnesota v. Hanson, 468 N.W. 2d 77,78 (1991).

17. Kauffman v. Alabama, 620 So. 2d 90 (1993).

Bibliography

REVIEW OF HUMAN STUDIES ON MEDICAL USE OF MARIJUANA

SUMMARY:
HUMAN STUDIES ON MEDICAL USES OF MARIJUANA

Hundreds of studies have been done on the medical uses of cannabis since its introduction to Western medicine in the early nineteenth century. A review of the literature reveals over 65 human studies, most of them in the 1970s and early '80s.

- **The best-established medical use of smoked marijuana is as an antinauseant for cancer chemotherapy.** Marijuana's efficacy was demonstrated in studies by half a dozen states, involving hundreds of subjects. Most research has found smoked marijuana superior to oral THC (Marinol). Many oncologists are currently recommending marijuana to their patients.

- **Marijuana is widely used to treat nausea and appetite loss associated with AIDS, but the government has blocked research in this area.** Studies have shown that marijuana helps improve appetite, and Marinol has been FDA-approved for treatment of AIDS wasting syndrome. Nearly 10,000 PWAs were reported to be using marijuana through the San Francisco Cannabis Buyers' Club. However, the government has blocked efforts by Dr. Donald Abrams of the University of California at San Francisco, to proceed with an FDA-approved study of marijuana and AIDS wasting syndrome, by refusing to grant him access to research marijuana. Research is badly needed on the relative merits of smoked and oral marijuana versus Marinol.

- **There is much evidence, largely anecdotal, that marijuana is useful as an anti-convulsant** for spinal injuries, multiple sclerosis, epilepsy, and other diseases. Similar evidence suggests marijuana may be useful as an **analgesic** for chronic pain from cancer and migraine as well as for rheumatism and a variety of autoimmune diseases. There is a conspicuous lack of controlled studies in this area; further research is needed.

• **Cannabidiol, a constituent of natural marijuana not found in Marinol, appears to have distinctive therapeutic value** as an anti-convulsant and hypnotic, and to counteract acute anxiety reactions caused by THC.

• **It has been established that marijuana reduces intraocular pressure,** the primary object of glaucoma therapy. Because of its psychoactivity, however, marijuana has not gained widespread acceptance in this application.

• **Many patients report using marijuana as a substitute for more addictive and harmful psychoactive drugs,** including prescription painkillers, opiates, and alcohol. Marijuana and Marinol have also been found useful as a **treatment for depression and mood disorders** in Alzheimer's and other patients. More research is needed.

Overview of Medical Marijuana Research

In its position paper, *Use of Marijuana as a "Medicine,"* the California Narcotics Officers Association refers to "10,000 studies . . . documenting the harmful physical and psychological effects of smoking marijuana." This myth has been effectively debunked in a letter to Dr. Lester Grinspoon from NIDA's marijuana research librarian at the University of Mississippi, Beverly Urbanek, who writes, "We are totally in the dark as to where the statement that there are 10,000 studies showing the negative impact of marijuana could have originated." She explains that while her library has some 12,000 citations on cannabis, they cover a broad spectrum of economic, legal, horticultural, enforcement, and other non-health issues, and are not categorized according to negative or positive effects.

Pursuing the issue further, it is possible to enumerate an impressive number of studies on marijuana's therapeutic uses. There is no space here to list or summarize all of them. The book *Cannabinoids as Therapeutic Agents*, edited by Dr. Raphael Mechoulam (CRC, 1986), includes copious references to research articles on cannabis' pharmacological effects, as follows:

Pharmacohistory of Cannabis Sativa — 90 references
Therapeutic Potential of Cannabinoids in Neurological Disorders — 155
Ocular Effects — 70
Cannabinoids as Antiemetics in Cancer — 91
Cannabinoids and Analgesia — 136
Bronchodilator Action of Cannabinoids — 67
Of course, there are some duplications, and by no means all of these 609 references actually detail medicinal benefits of marijuana, but it certainly seems reasonable to estimate that **there have been hundreds of studies on the medical use of marijuana.**

HUMAN STUDIES

Here is a summary of the *human* clinical and epidemiological studies on marijuana's therapeutic applications. We have not attempted to detail the great bulk of research, which consists of animal and in vitro studies whose relevance to human health is less clear. However, we have tried to include all human studies reported in the recent medical literature.

ANTINAUSEANT FOR CANCER CHEMOTHERAPY

This is by far the best-substantiated use of medical marijuana.

There have been at least 31 human studies of marijuana and/or oral THC for cancer chemotherapy,[1] beginning with the pathbreaking work of Sallan and Zinberg, the first modern study of medical marijuana.[2]

This doesn't include the studies in which the sponsors of Marinol got it FDA-approved as "safe and effective" for cancer chemotherapy.

Smoked marijuana was shown to be an effective antinauseant in six different state-sponsored clinical studies:[3] New Mexico (250 patients),[4] New York (199 patients),[5] California (98),[6] Tennessee (27),[7] Georgia (119),[8] and Michigan (165).[9]

Smoked marijuana was found to be superior to oral THC in the New Mexico and Tennessee studies, with efficacy rates of 90%. In New York and Tennessee, it was effective in patients who had not been helped by

Marinol. In Michigan, patients found smoked marijuana preferable to a conventional prescription antinauseant (Torecan). Other researchers have also reported smoked marijuana to be superior to THC.[10]

The California study was the least satisfactory, being highly biased toward oral THC (2000 patients were given oral THC, versus only 98 for marijuana): still, it found that marijuana was effective in 59% of patients, versus 57% for oral THC; however, 30% rated oral THC "highly effective," versus only 17% for marijuana. This is the only state study showing smoked marijuana inferior to Marinol.[11]

A survey of oncologists by Doblin and Kleiman reported that 44% of 1035 respondents had recommended marijuana to their patients (54% favored making it a prescription drug).[12]

GLAUCOMA

It is generally accepted — by the National Academy of Sciences and others — that **marijuana/THC reduces intraocular pressure (IOP)**, the basic aim of anti-glaucoma therapy.[13]

This was shown in a series of experiments by Robert S. Hepler of UCLA, arising from research aimed at finding out whether marijuana dilated pupils.[14] Hepler found a "statistically significant" drop in IOP in 429 subjects treated with marijuana or THC; a subset of 29 patients showed continued benefits during 94 days of treatment, with no signs of tolerance.[15] The effects of THC/marijuana in reducing IOP were explored in a half dozen other studies.[16]

Nonetheless, ophthalmologists have been reluctant to accept marijuana/THC because of its high psychoactivity. Efforts to develop topical cannabinoid eye drops as a nonpsychoactive alternative have so far proven unfruitful.

The California Research Advisory Panel established a glaucoma research protocol under its cannabis research program of 1979–89, after finding interest in marijuana in its survey of ophthalmologists. The program flopped: only nine patients were treated; all chose to take Marinol instead of marijuana, and and all eventually abandoned treatment.

AIDS AND APPETITE STIMULATION

There have been no clinical studies on the use of marijuana for AIDS. Of course, one reason for this is that the government has blocked the study by Dr. Donald Abrams at the University of California at San Francisco by denying him access to research marijuana.

Nonetheless, Marinol has been FDA-approved as an appetite stimulant for treating AIDS wasting syndrome.[17]

There is also an extensive literature on smoked marijuana and appetite stimulation, including four clinical studies in which marijuana enhanced food intake and weight gain.[18]

Medical marijuana is widely used by AIDS patients. Eighty percent of the SF Cannabis Buyers' Club's 11,000 customers are said to be PWAs.[19] A recent survey of HIV-positive gays in Australia found that one quarter were using marijuana therapeutically.[20]

Many AIDS patients prefer smoked marijuana to oral THC, because of its quickness of action, the ease of controlling the dose, and the absence of side effects. In addition to appetite stimulation, many AIDS patients use marijuana for pain associated with neuropathy, shingles, and so on.

An important concern connected with smoked marijuana that critics emphasize is the danger of respiratory infection in AIDS patients caused by smoking. In particular, critics have cited a worrisome study by Caiaffa et al.,[21] showing a twofold increase in the rate of pneumonocystis carinii pneumonia (PCP) among HIV-positive injection-drug users who smoke illegal drugs (88% marijuana, 26% cocaine, 9% crack cocaine). The study has a few problems, notably that almost all the subjects also smoked cigarettes; therefore, it's difficult to say whether the PCP was really due to marijuana.

In any case, these problems can be avoided by taking marijuana orally, which many AIDS patients in fact do. It's not clear whether oral marijuana has more medical benefits than Marinol, though it could certainly be more economical.

Another problem that critics like to emphasize is the supposed threat to PWAs posed by the immunosuppressive properties of marijuana. Of course, these objections apply equally well to oral THC, which has been approved for treatment of AIDS. Studies of THC's effects on immunity have been contradictory, and are not easy to interpret.[22] There are hints that THC might actually help stimulate the immune system in some ways.[23]

Epidemiological studies have found no relation between marijuana use and development of AIDS.[24] One recent study of 354 HIV-positive males actually found marijuana to be associated with a *decreased* rate of progression to AIDS, though the difference was not significant when adjusted for parameters reflecting the initial health of the study's subjects.[25]

MUSCLE SPASTICITY, MS, EPILEPSY, AND SPINAL INJURIES

The treatment of convulsions was the first major application of cannabis in Western medicine, attested by 19th-century authorities such as Dr. William O'Shaughnessy, the Ohio State Medical Committee, and Dr. John Russell Reynolds (who prescribed it to Queen Victoria for menstrual cramps).[26] Although it is well authenticated in traditional practice, modern research into this application has been scant, except for animal studies.

Altogether, there appear to be:

Five human case studies, involving a total of **eight patients,** in which **marijuana** was reported to be useful for **epilepsy, multiple sclerosis, injury, and Tourette's syndrome;**[27]

One study in which five out of eight **spinal cord injury** patients reported benefits from **marijuana;**[28]

Three more studies of **THC for multiple sclerosis** (total: 30 patients), in which benefits tended to be more subjective than objectively measurable;[29]

One case study of **THC for spinal cord injury;**[30]

Two clinical studies in which **cannabidiol (CBD),** a component of natural marijuana not found in Marinol, was found beneficial for grand mal epilepsy (15 subjects, double-blind controls)[31] and **dystonia** (five patients, no controls).[32]

One study in which a THC-related cannabinoid benefited two out of five severely epileptic children;[33]

One **survey of 308 epileptic patients**, which found that **marijuana** use appeared to delay the first onset of complex partial seizures.[34]

One **survey of 43 spinal cord injury patients** at VA hospitals, which found that 56% smoked **marijuana** and 88% reported that it reduced their muscle spasms.[35]

There have also been a couple of **negative studies**, finding no benefits of marijuana for Parkinsonism[36] or CBD for Huntington's chorea.[37] Paradoxically, marijuana/THC has been reported to exacerbate spasticity or epilepsy on occasion, perhaps because of a rebound effect.

In a purported recent **negative study on marijuana and multiple sclerosis**, Dr. Harry Greenberg et al., at the University of Michigan, reported that marijuana impaired posture and balance in patients with spastic MS.[38] This should come as no surprise, since marijuana/THC also impairs balance in normal patients. In any event, MS patients don't use marijuana for posture/balance, but to reduce tremors and pain.

CANNABIDIOL

There is considerable evidence from animal studies that CBD has distinctive anticonvulsant properties not found in THC.[39]

In addition, there is evidence that **CBD can reduce the risk of panic reactions associated with THC**. A study by Zuardi found that CBD reduces the anxiety-stimulating effects of THC, a leading cause of adverse reactions to Marinol.[40] This may be a reason why many patients prefer natural cannabis.

A controlled study of 15 insomniacs found that CBD helped subjects sleep better.[41]

ANALGESIA & PAIN

Many patients report using marijuana for some form of pain relief. Cannabis was used as an analgesic from ancient times through the nineteenth century. As we have mentioned, this use declined with the introduction of more potent opiates, such as injected morphine. Cannabis continued to be regarded as a drug of choice for migraine into the Twentieth century.

Modern research is scant. Animal studies have tended to show analgesic effects, but human studies have conflicted more:

In a preliminary study by R. J. Noyes, patients reported that marijuana relieved **migraine, menstrual cramps, postsurgical pain**. [42]

In a follow-up, Noyes found that oral THC relieved **chronic pain** in 10 **cancer patients**.[43]

In a second follow-up with 36 cancer patients, **THC was as effective as codeine**, but had more side effects.[44]

Two other studies found marijuana and THC effective in reducing experimentally induced pain.[45]

One study reported that three patients began to experience **migraines** only after giving up marijuana.[46]

Negative results have also been reported:

One study failed to find THC benefical for cancer pain, though it did help with depression and loss of appetite.[47]

One study found THC useless for artificially induced pain.[48]

One study found marijuana *increased* sensitivity to electrically induced pain.[49]

One study found CBD useless for neuropathic pain (10 patients).[50]

INFLAMMATORY DISEASES

Marijuana is used by many patients for a wide variety of diseases characterized by inflammation. These include arthritis, rheumatism, lupus, multiple sclerosis, colitis, Crohn's disease, inflammatory gastritis, scleroderma, endometriosis, psoriasis, and pruritis. These diseases are thought to be autoimmune in nature. It is possible that the supposed immuno suppressive properties of cannabis are beneficial for such conditions.

Unfortunately, there have been no clinical studies of this phenomenon. However, a variety of animal and laboratory studies have shown that cannabinoids have anti-inflammatory properties.[51] One mouse study even suggested that a non-cannabinoid ingedient of marijuana may be involved.[52]

ASTHMA

Although this isn't (and shouldn't be) an indication of choice for medical marijuana, three human studies have shown that smoking marijuana produces bronchodilation, thereby relieving asthma attacks.[53] Two other studies confirmed the same effects with THC.[54] Efforts to develop a smokeless THC inhaler have proven unsuccessful.

DEPRESSION & MENTAL ILLNESS

Opponents of medical marijuana, such as the CNOA, have charged that marijuana causes depression. In fact, marijuana is more often used to treat depression; hence its notoriety as a euphoriant. Human studies have been inconsistent. One study found that marijuana helped relieve depression in cancer patients;[55] another found no benefit for clinical depression.[56]

A survey of 79 mental patients found that those who used marijuana reported relief from depression, anxiety, insomnia, and physical discomfort, as well as fewer hospitalizations;[57] a second survey also found fewer hospitalizations in schizophrenics who used marijuana.[58] Some psychiatrists are currently prescribing Marinol for depression.

A recent pilot study by the Unimed Corporation found that Marinol helped relieve mood disturbances and anorexia in 12 Alzheimer's patients.[59]

ALCOHOLISM & DRUG DEPENDENCE

Cannabis is often used as a substitute for other, more dangerous drugs, including prescription narcotics, opiates, and alcohol. Cannabis has been proposed as a treatment for alcoholism as well as for opiate addiction.[60] However, a single controlled study of cannabis to treat alcoholics proved unsuccessful.[61] There is some epidemiological evidence that substitution of marijuana for alcohol and other drugs tends to reduce drug abuse and accident costs.[62] Many cannabis buyers' club members say they use marijuana as a substitute for prescription narcotics.[63]

VIOLENCE

Many opponents absurdly charge that marijuana aggravates violence. To this, the best answer is that of the National Academy of Science in *Marihuana and Health* (1982, p. 128):

"Both retrospective and experimental studies in human beings have failed to yield evidence that marijuana use leads to increased aggression. Most of these studies suggest quite the contrary effect. Marijuana appears to have a sedative effect, and it may reduce somewhat the intensity of angry feelings and the probability of interpersonal aggressive behavior."

REFERENCES

Raphael Mechoulam, ed., *Cannabinoids as Therapeutic Agents* (CRC Press, Boca Raton), 1986.

Lester Grinspoon and James Bakalar, *Marihuana, the Forbidden Medicine* (Yale University Press), 1993.

Sidney Cohen and Richard Stillman, eds., *The Therapeutic Potential of Marihuana* (Plenum, NY), 1975.

Tod Mikuriya, *Marijuana Medical Papers* (Medicomp Press, Berkeley), 1973.

Robert Randall, *Marijuana, Medicine and the Law* (Galen Press, Washington, D.C.), 1989 (2 volumes).

National Academy of Sciences, *Marijuana and Health*, Report of the Institute of Medicine (National Academy Press), 1982. (NAS Report)

Laura Murphy and Andrzej Bartke, eds., *Marijuana/Cannabinoids: Neurobiology and Neurophysiology* (CRC Press, Boca Raton), 1992.

M. C. Braude and S. Szara, eds., *Pharmacology of Marihuana*, NIDA Monograph (Raven Press, NY), 1976 (2 volumes).

REFERENCES ON GLAUCOMA

Martin Adler and Ellen Geller, "Ocular Effects of Cannabinoids," Chapter 3 in Mechoulam.

Chapters 4–6 "Ophthalmic Effects," in Cohen and Stillman.

REFERENCES ON ANTICONVULSANT PROPERTIES

P. Consroe and R. Sandyk, "Potential Role of Cannabinoids for Therapy of Neurological Disorders," Chapter 12 in Murphy and Bartke.

Paul Consroe and Stuart Snider, "Therapeutic Potential of Cannabinoids in Neurological Disorders," Chapter 2 in Mechoulam.

REFERENCES ON ANALGESIA

Mark Segal, "Cannabinoids and Analgesia," Chapter 6 in Mechoulam.

END NOTES

1. Includes (a) 25 studies of oral THC listed in M. Levitt, "Cannabinoids as Antiemetics in Cancer Chemotherapy," in Mechoulam, p. 73; (b) 6 state studies of marijuana listed below.

2. S. Sallan, N. Zinberg, and E. Frei, "Antiemetic effect of delta-9-tetrahydro-cannabinol in patients receiving cancer chemotherapy," *New England Journal of Medicine* 295: 795 (1975).

3. For a summary, see Robert Randall, ed., *Marijuana, Medicine and the Law*, vol . 2 (Galen Press, Washington D.C.), 1989, 36ff.

4. New Mexico: 250 patients; 90% relieved; only 3 adverse reactions (all with THC): testimony of Daniel Dansak, M.D. in Robert Randall, ed., *Marijuana, Medicine and the Law*, vol. 1, 125–33; vol. 2, 36–8.

5. New York: 199 patients evaluated; all had failed with previous antinauseants (some also failed with THC); marijuana 89.7%–100% effective at 3 hospitals. ACT Official State Reports, vol. II, Exhibit 15, "Evaluation of the Antiemetic Properties of Inhalation Marijuana in Cancer Patients Receiving Chemotherapy Treatment," NY Dept of Health, Office of Public Health, Chapter 810, Laws of 1980 Article 33-A, Public Health Law, September 1981; ACT Exhibit 16-C, "Impressions from the National Conference on the Therapeutic Applications of Cannabinoids." Cited in Randall, vol. 2, 46–54.

6. California: 98 patients received marijuana; 59% found it effective against strong emetics; 57% of 257 patients found THC-only effective; 17% rated marijuana "very effective" versus 30% for THC. *Cannabis Therapeutic Research Program*, Report to the Cal. Legislature by California Research Advisory Panel, Jan. 1989. See also Randall, vol. 2, 55–63.

7. Tennessee: 27 patients evaluared of 43 who had failed other therapy, including THC; 90.4% successful on marijuana; 66.7% on oral THC. ACT Official State Reports, vol. II, Exhibit 17, *Annual Report: Evaluation of Marijuana and Tetrahydrocannabinol in the Treatment of Nausea and/or Vomiting Associated with Cancer Therapy Unresponsive to Conventional Antiemetic Therapy: Efficacy and Toxicity*, Board of Pharmacy, State of Tennessee, July 1983. Cited in Randall, vol. 2, 55.

8. Georgia: 119 evaluable patients; THC or marijuana 73% effective; marijuana
    had 6 adverse reactions from smoke intolerance; THC had 6 panic reactions.
    Michael H. Kuttner, *Evaluation of the Use of Both Marijuana and THC in
    Cancer Patients for the Relief of Nausea and Vomiting Associated with Cancer
    Chemotherapy After Failure of Conventional Anti-Emetic Therapy: Efficacy and
    Toxicity*, report for the Composite State Board of Medical Examiners, Georgia
    Dept. of Health, by researchers at Emory University 1/20/83. Cited in
    Randall, vol. 2, 38–43.

9. Michigan: Randomized crossover, marijuana versus Torecan; 165 patients;
    marijuana 71% effective — similar to Torecan, but patients preferred marijua-
    na. ACT Official State Reports, vol. II, Exhibit 9, *Evaluation of Marijuana as
    an Antiemetic in Patients Being Treated with Cancer Chemotherapy*, Protocol
    Trial A, IND # 17-193. Cited in Randall, vol. 2, 43.

10. E.g., Sallan and Zinberg (cited in Randall, vol. 2, 35), and A.E. Chang et al.,
    "Delta-9-THC as an Antiemetic in Cancer Patients Receiving High-Dose
    Methotrexate: A Prospective Randomized Evaluation," *Annals of Internal
    Medicine* 91 (1979), 819-24.

11. For another study in which oral THC was found superior to smoked marijuana
    in 20 subjects, see M. Levitt et al., "Randomized double-blind comparison of
    delta-9-tetrahydrocannabinol (THC) and marijuana as chemotherapy
    antiemetics," *ASCO Abstracts*, 3: 94 (1984); cited in Mechoulam, 73.

12. Rick Doblin and Mark Kleiman, "Marihuana as Anti-emetic Medicine: A sur-
    vey of Oncologists' Attitudes and Experiences," Journal of Clinical Oncology
    9:1275–80 (1991).

13. NAS Report, *Marijuana and Health*, 140–142.

14. R. S. Hepler and I. R.Frank, "Marihuana smoking and intraocular pressure,"
    JAMA 217:1392 (1971). Hepler, R. S., Frank, I. M., and Ungerleider, J. T.
    "Pupillary constriction after marijuana smoking," *Am J Ophthalmol.* 74:
    1185–90, 1972. Hepler, R. S., Frank, I. M., and Petrus, R., "Ocular effects of
    marihuana smoking," in Braude and Szara, vol. 2: 815–24 (Raven, NY), 1976.

15. Robert S. Hepler and Robert J. Petrus, "Experiences with Administration of
    Marihuana to Glaucoma Patients," Chapter 5 (63–94) in Cohen and
    Stillman.

16. Shapiro, D., "The ocular mainfestations of the cannabinols," *Ophthalmologica* 1974 168:366-9; Purnell, W. D. and Gregg, J. M. "Delta-9 THC, euphoria and intraocular pressure in man," *Annals of Ophthalmology*, July 1975; Greeen, K. and Podos, S. M. "Antagonism of arachidonic acid-induced ocular effects by delta-THC" *Investigative Ophthalmology*, June 1974; Flom, M. C., Adams, A. J. and Jones, R. T., "Marijuana smoking and reduced pressure in human eyes: drug action or epiphenomenon?", *Invest. Ophtalmol.*, 14:52 (1975); Cooler, P. and Gregg, J. M. "Effect of delta-9-THC on introacoular pressure in humans," *South Med J.* 70: 954, 1977; Paul Cooler and John Gregg, "The effect of delta-9-THC on intraocular pressure in humans," Chapter 6 in Cohen and Stillman; Merritt, J. C., et al., "Oral delta-9-THC in heterogeneous glaucomas," *Ann. Ophthalmol.*, 12:947 (1980); Perez-Reyes, M. et al., "Intravenous administration of cannabinoids and intraocular pressure," in Braude and Szara, 829; "Jones, R., Benowitz, N., and Herning, R. I., "Clinical relevance of cannabis tolerance and dependence," *J Clin Pharmacol*, 21:143S (1981).

17. T. F. Plasse, R. W. Gorter, S. H. Krasnow, et al., "Recent Clinical Experience with Dronabinol," *Pharmacology, Biochemistry and Behavior* 40 (1991), 695–700.

18. L. E. Hollister, "Hunger and Appetite after Single Doses of Marihuana, Alcohol, and Dextroamphetamine," *Clinical Pharmacology and Therapeutics* 12 (Jan.–Feb. 1971), 44–9.

    27 marihuana users and 10 controls — gained weight in hospital ward: Greenberg et al., "Effects of Marihuana Use on Body Weight and Caloric Intake in Humans," *Journal of Pscyhopharmacology* (Berlin) 49 (1976), 79–84.

    9 subjects gained weight smoking marihuana rather than placebo cigarettes: R. W. Foltin et al., "Behavioral Analysis of Marijuana Effects on Food Intake in Humans," *Pharmacology, Biochemistry and Behavior* 25 (1986), 577–82.

    6 subjects increased caloric intake 40% over 13 days: R. W. Foltin et al., "Effects of smoked marijuana on food intake and body weight in humans living in a residential laboratory," Appetite 1988: 11:1–14.

19. Personal communication.

20. 228 subjects: Prestage, Garrett, et al., "Use of Treatments and Health-Enhancement Behavior Among HIV-Positive Men in a Cohort of Homosexually-Active Men," XI International Converence on AIDS, Vancouver, B.C., Canada, July 1996.

21. W. T. Caiaffa et al., "Drug Smoking, Pneumonocystis Carinii Pneumonia, and Immunosuppression Increase Risk of Bacterial Pneumonia in Human Immunodeficiency Virus-seropositive Injection Drug Users," *Am J Respir Crit Care Med*, 150: 1493–8 (1994).

22. Leo Hollister, "Marijuana and Immunity," *Journal of Psychoactive Drugs* 20(1): 3–8 (Jan./Mar. 1988).

23 One study of 10 healthy subjects found significantly higher T-cell counts after exposure to marijuana: D. Tashkin, "Cannabis 1977," *Ann. Intern. Med.* 89:539–49 (1978).

   Recent lab studies have variously found that THC (1) decreases interleukin-6, while increasing tumor necrosis factor-alpha: S. C. Shivers et al., "Delta-9-THC modulates IL-1 bioactivity in human monocyte/macrophage cell lines," *Life Sciences* 54(17) 1281–9 (1994); or (2) inhibits TNF-alpha: H Friedman et al., "Marijuana, receptors and immunomodulation," *Advances in Experimental Medicine and Biology* 373: 103–113 (1995); or (3) stimulates production of interleukin 2 in rats: Susan Pross at the University of South Florida, Tampa (personal communication).

24. Richard A. Kaslow et al., "No Evidence for a Role of Alcohol or Other Psychoactive Drugs in Accelerating Immunodeficiency in HIV-1 Positive Individuals," JAMA 261:3424–9 (June 16, 1989); M. S. Ascher et al., "Does drug use cause AIDS?," *Nature* 36: 103–4 (March 11, 1993).

25. Di Franco et al., "The Lack of Association of Marijuana and Other Recreational Drugs with Progression to AIDS in the SFMHS," XI International Conference on AIDS, Vancouver, B.C., Canada, July 1996.

26. O'Shaughnessy, W.B., "On the Preparation of the Indian Hemp or Gunja," (1839), *Report of the Ohio State Medical Committee on Cannabis Indica* (1860) and J. R. Reynolds, "Therapeutical Uses and Toxic Effects of Cannabis Indica," in Tod H. Mikuriya, ed., *Marijuana: Medical Papers*.

27. 1 MS patient: Clifford,D. B., "THC for Tremor in Multiple Sclerosis," *Annals of Neurology* 13 (1983) 669-71.

   1 MS patient: Meinck, H. M., Schlone, F. W., and Conrad, B., "Effects of Cannabinoids on Spasticity and Ataxia in Multiple Sclerosis," *Journal of Neurology* 236 (1989), 120–2.

   1 epileptic: Consroe, P., Wood, G. C., and Buchsbaum, H., "Anticonvulsant Nature of Marihuana Smoking," JAMA 234 (1975), 306–7.

3 Tourette's cases: Sandyk, R., and Awerbuch, G., "Marijuana and Tourette's Syndrome," *J Clin Psychopharmacol*. 8: 444 (1988).

1 MS, 1 injury patient: Petro, D. J., "Marijuana as a therapeutic agent for muscle spasm or spasticity," *Psychosomatics* 221: 81 (1980).

28. Dunn, M. and Davis, R., "The perceived effects of marijuana on spinal cord injured males," Paraplegia 12:175 (1974).

29. 13 MS patients — THC had subjective, but not objective effects: Ungerleider, T., et al., "Delta-9-THC in the treatment of spasticity associated with multiple sclerosis," *Adv Alcohol Substance Abuse* 7:39 (1987).

5 of 8 MS patients had subjective benefits, 2 of 8 objective: Clifford, D. B., "Thc for tremor in multiple sclerosis," *Ann Neurol* 13:669 (1983).

9 MS patients double-blind reduced spasms; also 3 with tonic spasms: Petro, D. J., and Ellenberger, C., "Treatment of human spasticity with delta-9-THC," *J Clin Pharmacol* 21: 413S, 1981.

30. Maurer, M., et al., "Delta-9-THC Shows Antispastic and Analgesic Effects in a Single Case Double-Blind Trial," *European Archives of Psychiatry and Clincial Neuroscience* 240 (1990) 1–4.

31. Cunha, J. M. et al., "Chronic Administration of Cannabidiol to Healthy Volunteers and Epileptic Patients," *Pharmacology* 21 (1980) 175–85.

32. Consroe, P. and Sandyk, R., "Open label evaluation of cannabidiol in dystonic movement disorders," *Int J Neurosci*, 30: 277 (1986).

33. Davis, J. P. and Ramsey, H. H., "Antiepileptic Action of Marijuana-active Substances," *Federation Proceedings* 8 (1949), 284–5.

34. Ellison, W. R. et al., "Complex partial seizure symptoms affected by marijuana abuse," *Journal of Clinical Psychiatry* 51: 439 (1990).

35. Malec, J., Harvey, R. F., and Cayner, J. J., "Cannabis Effect on Spasticity in Spinal Cord Injury," *Archives of Physical and Medical Rehabilitation* 63 (March 87), 116–8.

36. Frankel, J. P. et al, "Marijuana for Parkinsonian tremor," *J. Neurol. Neurosurg. Psychiatry* 53:436 (1990).

37. Consroe, P. et al., "Controlled clinical trial of cannabidiol in Huntington's disease," *Pharmacol Biochem Behav* 40: 701 (1991).

38. Greenberg, Harry S. et al., "Short-term effects of smoking marijuana on balance in patients with multiple sclerosis and normal volunteers," *Clin Pharmacol Therap* March 1994: 55:324–8.

39. Consroe, P., and Sandyk, R., "Potential Role of Cannabinoids for Therapy of Neurological Disorders," Chapter 12 in Murphy and Bartke, 482–3.
40. 8 human subjects: Zuardi, A. W. et al., "Action of cannabidiol on the anxiety and other effects produced by delta-9-THC in normal subjects," *Psychopharmacology* 76: 245–50 (1982).
41. Carlini, E. A. and Cunha, J. M., "Hypnotic and Antiepileptic Effects of Cannabidiol," *Journal of Clinical Pharmacology* 21: 4175–275 (1981).
42. Noyes, Jr., R. J. and Baram, D. A., "Cannabis analgesia," *Compr Psychiatry* 15:531 (1973).
43. Noyes, R. J., et al., "The Analgesic Effect of Delta-9-THC," *Journal of Clinical Pharmacology* 14 (Feb./Mar. 1975) 139–43.
44. Noyes, R. J., et al., "The Analgesic Properties of Delta-9-THC and Codeine," *Clinical Pharmacology and Therapeutics* 18 (1975) 84–9.
45. Analgesic effects on thumbnail test: Milstein, S. L. et al., "Marijuana-produced Changes in Pain Tolerance: Experienced and Non-experienced Subjects," *International Pharmacopsychiatry* 10:177–182 (1975);
    Four subjects tested with thermal pain: Zeidenberg et al., "Effects of oral administration of Delta-9-THC on memory, speech and perception of thermal stimulation": *Compr. Psychiatry* 14:549 (1973).
46. El-Mallakh, R. S., "Marijuana and migraine," *Headache* 27, 442 (1989).
47. Regelson et al., "Delta-9-THC as an effective antidepressant and appetite-stimulating agent in advanced cancer patients," in Braude and Szara, pp. 763–76.
48. Raft, D. et al., "Effects of intravenous THC on experimental surgical pain," *Clin Pharmacol Ther* 21:26 (1977).
49. Hill et al., "Marijuana and pain," *J Pharmacol Exp Ther* 188:415 (1974).
50. Lindstrom, P. et al., "Lack of effect of cannabidiol in sustained neuropathic [pain]," *Marijuana '87*, Int. Conf. on Cannabis, Melbourne, 1987.
51. Barret, M. L. et al., "Isolation from Cannabis sativa L. of Cannflavon — a novel inhibitor of prostaglandin production," *Biochem. Pharmacol.* 34: 2019 (1985); Burstein, S. H. et al., "Antagonism to the actions of platelet activating factor by a nonpsychoactive cannabinoid," *J Pharmacol. Exp. Therap.* 251: 531–5 (1989); Sofia, R. D., "Antiedemic and analgesic properties of delta-9-THC compared with three other drugs," *Eur. J. Pharamacol.* 41: 705–9 (1989).

52. Formukong, E. A., Evans, A. T., and Evans, F. J., "Analgesic and antiinflammatory activity of constitutents of Cannabis sativa L." *Inflammation* 12#4: 361 (1988).

53. Tashkin, D. P., Shapiro, B. J. and Frank, I. M., "Acute effects of smoked marijuana and oral delta-9-THC on specific airway conductance in asthmatic subjects," *Am Rev Respir Dis* 109: 420–8 (1974); Tashkin, D. P. et al., "Effects of smoked marijuana in experimentally induced asthma," *Am Rev Respir Dis* 112:377-86 (1975); Vachon, L. et al., "Bronchial effects of marijuana smoke in asthma," in Braude and Szara, 777ff.

54. Tashkin, D. P., Shapiro, B. J., and Frank, I. M., "Acute Pulmonary Physicologic Effects of Smoked Marihuana and Oral Delta-9-THC in Healthy Young Men," *New England Journal of Medicine*, 289: 336-41 (1973). ; Vachon, L., Robins, A., and Gaensler, E. A., "Airways Response to Aerosolized Delta-9-THC: Preliminary Report," Chapter 8 in Cohen and Stillman.

55. Regelson et al., "Delta-9-THC as an effective antidepressant and appetite-stimulating agent in advanced cancer patients," in Braude and Szara, 763–76.

56. Eight controlled depression patients: Kotin et al., "Delt-9-THC in depressed patients," *Arch Gen Psychiatry* 28:345-8, 1973.

57. Warner, Richard et al., "Substance Use Among the Mentally Ill," *American Journal of Orthopsychiatry*, Jan. 1994.

58. Meuser, K. T. et al., "Prevalence of substance abuse in schizophrenia," *Schizophrenia Bulletin* 16: 31–56 (1990).

59. Study by Dr. Ladislav Volicer of Boston University: press release by Unimed Pharmaceuticals, Buffalo Grove, IL, July 29, 1996.

60. Tod Mikuriya, "Cannabis Substitution: An Adjunctive Therapeutic Tool in the Treatment of Alcoholism," *Medical Times* 98 #4: 187–91 (1970); reprinted in Mikuriya, *Marijuana Medical Papers*; also, Chaim Rosenberg, "The Use of Marihuana in the treatment of alcoholism," Chapter 13 in Cohen and Stillman.

61. Rosenberg, C. M. et al., "Cannabis in the treatment of alcoholism," *J Stud. Alcohol* 39:1955-8 (1978).

62. Chaloupka, Frank and Laixuthal, Adit, "Do Youths Substitute Alcohol and Marijuana? Some Econometric Evidence," *National Bureau of Economic Research Working Paper No. 4662*, Cambridge, MA, 1993; Karyn Model, "The

Effect of Marijuana Decriminalization on Hospital Emergency Room Episodes," *Journal of the American Statistical Association* 88:423 737–47 (1993) ; see also Passell, Peter, "Less Marijuana, More Alcohol?" *The New York Times,* June 17, 1992, C2.

63. Mikuriya, Tod, personal communication.

—*by Dale H. Gieringer, Ph.D.*

August 26, 1996

California NORML

2215-R Market St. #278, San Francisco, CA 94114

(415) 563-5858 / canorml@igc.apc.org

This document available on http://www.norml.org/canorml

Glossary

AMA — American Medical Association

Analgesic — A medication that reduces or eliminates pain.

Antiemetic — Treatment for severe nausea and vomiting.

CAMP — Campaign Against Marijuana Planting

CBC — Cannabichrome

CBD — Cannabidiol

CBL — Cannabicyclol

CBN — Cannabinol

CBG — Cannbigerol

CBT — Cannabitriol

CFS — Chronic Fatigue Syndrome

CO_2 — Carbon Dioxide, an odorless, colorless gas.

Cannabinoid — Any of the class of chemicalsunique to the cannabis plant, including THC, CBC, CBD, some of which have medicinal and psychoactive properties.

Cannabis — The botanical name for marijuana.

DEA — Drug Enforcement Administration

Delta-8-THC — Close relative of Delta-9 (THC) with some what less psychoactive potency.

Delta-9-THC — THC, the main psychoactive ingredient in marijuana.

FDA — Food and Drug Administration

Glands — Very potent part of marijuana buds.

HPS — High-Pressure-Sodium

Hashish — Concentrated cannabis resin.

Hydroponic — Cultivation of plants in nutrient solution rather than in soil.

IOP — Intraocular Pressure; fluid pressure in the eye.

Indica — Strain of marijuana from the Afghan region.

Kief — Unpressed hashish.

MAPS — Multidisciplinary Association for Psychedelic Studies

MH — Metal Halide

MPP — Marijuana Policy Project

Marinol — Synthetic drug which contains pure THC.

NHTSA — National Highway Transportation Safety Administration

NIDA — National Institute on Drug Abuse

NORML — National Organization for the Reform of Marijuana Laws

Oncologist — The branch of medicine that deals with tumors, including study of development, diagnosis, treatment, and prevention of cancer.

Opiates — Any of various sedative narcotics containing opium or one or more of its natural or synthetic derivatives.

P — Phosphorous

pH — A measure of the acidity or alkalinity of a solution, numerically equal to 7 for neutral solutions, increasing with increasing alkalinity and decreasing with increasing acidity. The pH scale commonly in use ranges from 0 to 14.

PWA — People With AIDS

REM — Rapid-Eye-Movement (sleep type associated with dreaming)

Sativa — Strain of marijuana from India and Thailand.

Schedule 1 — Federal classification of a drug that says it has no medical use and can't be prescribed by a doctor.

Schedule 2 — Federal classification of a drug that means it can be prescribed by doctors for limited purposes.

Sinsemila — Seedless marijuana.

THC — Tetrahdrocannabinol, the main active ingredient in marijuana.

Tincture — An alcohol solution of a nonvolatile medicine.

UCLA — University of California Los Angeles

VA — Veterans Administration

Waterpipe — Draws smoke through a water filter.

Index

Also available at your local bookstore:

Marijuana Grower's Handbook
by Ed Rosenthal
The most helpful reference book around for indoor and greenhouse cultivation. Contains over 100 photos showing the steps to maintaining a high yield garden. Explains hydroponic growing in-depth, and covers any situation that could come up during the growth cycle.
232 pages, $19.95 ISBN# 0-932551-02-5

Marihuana Reconsidered
by Dr. Lester Grinspoon, M.D.
Back in print! First published by Harvard University Press in 1971, this is still the most comprehensive assessment of marihuana and its place in society. Noted psychiatrist Dr. Lester Grinspoon pulverizes the arguments that keep marijuana illegal. Updated with a new introduction by the author who still believes the most dangerous thing about smoking marihuana is getting caught.
500 pages, $19.95 ISBN# 0-932551-13-0

Marijuana Question? Ask Ed
by Ed Rosenthal
The Encyclopedia of Marijuana, this book contains everything you ever wanted to know, from cultivation to inhaling. Organized for easy reference, it gives practical, hands-on advice. The author proclaims this as his most helpful book, because it's based on readers' questions.
300 pages, $19.95 ISBN# 0-932551-01-7

Or call 1-800-428-7825 Ext.102,
or online at www.quicktrading.com

Also available at your local bookstore:

Marijuana, The Law and You
by William Logan, Ed Rosenthal & Jeffrey Steinborn
Written for both the consumers and attorneys.
Shows you how to stay out of trouble and out of jail.
Find out:
* What the police look for;
* How to avoid suspicion;
* How to beat the rap.
This book shows proven courtroom strategies that have
saved clients thousands of years in jail time. For best
results, read before needed!

*"This excellent book does a thorough job of covering
key legal areas of interest to anyone who is busted for
possession or cultivation."*
—Nolo Press

*"This book, written by experienced criminal defense
lawyers will empower both attorneys and defendants
accused of marijuana offenses."*
—R. Fogelnest, President, National Association of
Criminal Defense Lawyers

218 pages, $24.95 ISBN# 0-932551-18-1

Or call 1-800-428-7825 Ext.102,
or online at www.quicktrading.com